i

Published by The Dot Wot
ABN: 57566837638

EDITION 1

ISBN: 978-0-9875801-3-9

Contents
    1. questions

Dear Reader,

I made a promise to my unborn daughter that
I would share my understanding of the world
with the world. My daughter and I have not
yet had this 'talk', it is a sneak-peak for
your eyes only. I hope it is worth a
cucumber sandwich or two of contemplation:
*You may be the buddy my little girl needs
one day.* Thank you.

mum, I blame you for this book.

Entropy: Is a worrying word; it worried me to use it. However, logic gave me an offer I could not refuse. Entropy is the degree of randomness in a system. It describes the redundant energy created as energy is used to do non-redundant stuff; it must increase. It is a law of thermodynamics and is the twig I tripped over that threw me down the rabbit hole. When you read the word 'entropy' imagine you throw a handful of stones into a pond. Picture the Universe expanding like the rings that form. The rings collide creating new waves and correlations as the energy spreads and is dispersed. Entropy is the 'leaking' of available energy as the ripples die. It is the thing that makes you, the Universe and everything instantaneously beautiful.

questions

Aoife: What question should I ask?

Dad: Who am I?

Aoife: Who am I?

Dad: Your name is Aoife, (ee-far) you are my daughter, I love you.

Aoife: Who are you?

Dad: I am your Dad. I come from an isolated place called tasmania, it was home. When I was young my uncle's ride on lawnmower had its own carpark at the pub - it is that kind of place.

Aoife: Is the world scary?

Dad: The perception of it can be. Perception is fuzzy and furry. By fuzzy I mean unexplainable and by furry, I mean illusionary; that can be scary.

Aoife: What is love?

Dad: Love creates beautiful problems and provides beautiful solutions at the same time in a never-ending, disconcerting, imperfectly closed loop. Love is a cascade; our hearts beat faster, we sweat and become less predictable. We feel love resides in the heart and that is a lie. Love is a survival tool; it primes me to protect you. You may wonder, my little one, how does it help humankind that love should be so befuddling? Like the universe, love is perfectly imperfect and constantly seeking an unattainable equilibrium. Therefore, do not try to balance the love equation. It is enough for it to be well-adjusted.

Aoife: What is the difference?

Dad: Adjusted means tolerant, tolerance needs perception. Balanced means equal; equilibrium requires time to stop. Nothing is equal in the universe. Perceive what 'you' are and be tolerant.

Aoife: Of myself?

Dad: Yes, of your *Self*. 'Self' refers to that part of you designed to enable social interaction. Persevere with your Self; it is your mind's means for telling a story of survival. Love is like a metal detector that Self uses to source connections that lead to baby-making. Directly or indirectly, this is the only motivation Self needs to engage love. Reflect: *Like searching for a feather in the dark, love is elusive and leaves you wondering - this feather better be worth it!*

Aoife: What does being 'in love' mean?

Dad: Nothing. Love is 'in' you. Coursing through your veins. Forcing your hormones to make your heart race and your capillaries open. Love is 'in' everything. It is a product of *your* autonomous processes. Therefore, own your impulses; they are *your* possession.

Aoife: Are there different types of love?

Dad: Yes, and yes. The universe is love. There is also the type of love you have for me which is something like the love a fungus has for its host. It is also a kind of practice-love. Then there is romantic love. Which is the main race. But the victory laps are performed by babies because they are loved unconditionally and will forget. So essentially love becomes love and its importance or intensity is relative. So, when you experience the end of love remember it is a cycle; you are meant to love again and again.

Aoife: What then is a soulmate?

Dad: A fiction. It is a type of emotional blackmail. Humans are inclined to idealise intangibles. For instance, we celebrate the anorexic model and the steroidal Adonis, and we nip, tuck and filter accordingly. We want to define an elusive notion of perfection so it may inspire us to approximate. They are 'statusments'; ideals that are intentionally unattainable. The truth is anorexia and steroid use can result in premature death. Likewise, the term soulmate describes an ideal version of love that is never attained regardless of how long a relationship appears to last.

Aoife: What is the key to lasting relationships?

Dad: Fall in love over and over again; reflect the cycles of nature. Renewal is essential. Be aware, love is reconstructed; after the imperfect destruction of it. Destruction is the puppet-master of rebirth; do not fear it. So, when love begins to renew meditate on it and accept that the renewal process is de-constructive. Respect

love, our species relies on it. So, love
love and what it does for others; seeing
your love enliven other people should be a
natural consequence of loving love. It
should not be the reason why you think love
exists. This gives love the priority it
deserves. Love comes before all, even the
soul; soul is a type of music.

Aoife: Can love be forever?

Dad: Love is always forever; it *is* the
universe. The only way you can truly love is
to remember love truly. Never forget the
loves you have had. Recall the moment it
started, the beginning of its end and the
regret. Enjoy the cacophony of elation and
pain: *it is the manifestation of the entropy
that must increase in a perfectly imperfect
universe.* You are made of hydrogen atoms
that are over 13 billion years old - love is
the Big Bang, the infinite.

Aoife: Who should I love?

Dad: Someone who never loses their keys and
finishes everything they start. People who
lose their keys have 'Mother' issues. People
who cannot finish what they start are
narcissistic. Narcissism involves the
display of behaviours that render the
strongest *social* 'reflection'.
Unfortunately, most worthwhile endeavours
require hours of tedious, lonely toil. The
narcissist will be good at 'announcing' the
start of something that is unlikely to be
finished because they are 'launch' addicted.
They fail to engage meaningfully.

Aoife: Keys?

Dad: People who lose their keys are seeking to be dependant; they *might* have attachment issues. They can be dangerous because the attachments they make later in life are unsophisticated and experienced obsessively.

Aoife: What is passion?

Dad: Passion is a mistake. The blood boils, redundancy eddies, distraction stalks you like butt ends at a train station. Passion gets people killed. Do not be passionate. You are best to be energised. Which means you must eat right, think right, and do not do anything unless you are willing to complete it.

Aoife: But I want to feel passionate about things.

Dad: Then feel passionate. But first let the 'things' energise you. The joy of creation is not the completion of the task it is the execution, and that needs energy; passion is only the bubbles in the Champagne. Passion can afford the cart but not the horse. Energy buys the horse first and uses entrepreneurial skills to get others to pay for the cart.

Aoife: What about trust?

Dad: When and where logic fails, sense resists and alarms sound you must trust. First you must trust your *Self*, especially when it seems irrational. Trust, in the first instance, that your instincts are meaningful. Everything is relative, even the safe keeping of your Self is measured relatively. Face the unknown with the excitement that only the potential to fail can give you and lean heavily on trust. It will be the source of pride that fortifies you against an unpredictable world designed impeccably to constantly reconstruct itself.

Aoife: Who should I trust?

Dad: Most people, blindly. In terms of love, you must trust. Do not love in protection mode, give yourself to love. You need not give yourself to others necessarily, be guarded as your senses determine. But give yourself to love and if love gives you loss be grateful for the gift. Trust is the weight you put on the barbell that is love. Load it, work it, grow love and trim regret, and be more than what you were and less than what you need to be. Love is, simultaneously, both a very personal possession and an open aspect of your Self. Accept love has no security, it will end. So, love as much as you can while it lasts; then move on. Reflect: *Like a neck tattoo in a foreign language, make sure the translation is accurate.*

Aoife: Should I always trust myself?

Dad: That depends. Is your *Self* healthy? Does it function well? Is it a good social negotiator? Self is a construct designed to enable social viability. Therefore, every social interaction is a chance for you to train and strengthen Self. So, trust that your Self can learn and call it a smile-generator: *If your sense of who you are is motivated by the desire to make others*

*thrive and laugh then your Self is worthy of
trust.*

Aoife: Should I pick a side?

Dad: Always. Be prepared however to be
wrong. If you pick the wrong side, then you
have an advantage. Not only do you get to
reflect on the poor choice you made and
determine why you made that choice. You will
also have the chance to abandon others with
whom you had developed affinity.
Experiencing the fragility of conditional
loyalty will harden you against blind
obedience. It also means you will find the
necessary breaking of many hearts easier.

Aoife: Would mum survive the zombie
apocalypse?

Dad: Probably not. But neither will you. The
kind of mutation that means humans would
turn into cannibalistic, blood-thirsty,
mindless monsters would be aggressively
adaptive and would find a way to infect
everyone. Our progression to zombie is the
end of the species. It is a self-
consummation mythology developed because we
have an unacknowledged fear of the finite
and the infinite. Or more specifically, a
reluctance to accept that the infinite
cannot *know* the finite. Your mum would
probably want to eat your brains, but the
feeling would be mutual.

Aoife: Should I be on social media?

Dad: Yes. It is important that you have
access to a selection of attitudes you can
selectively ignore. Think of social media as

a way of looking through a window to see the
obsessions of others who want to be like who
you want to be like, so you know how to be
only *like* them.

Aoife: Approximate, don't simulate?

Dad: Yes. Social media is an expression of
entropy, a valid and entirely inevitable
manifestation. It is a hybridisation of
spiritual understandings; at the centre of
its cacophony is a tangential homogenising
that seeks to consolidate our sense of
presence beyond our comprehension of it. In
this way, it acts like an alien that knows
itself as a confounding of correlations, and
it knows only itself. It, therefore, appears
to mirror notions of unity towards the
validation of community. Instant by instant
it displays a counterfeit of endeavour. This
redundancy is measured against a degree of
purposefulness that, instant by instant, is
as affective as it needs to be. There is no
end, however, to its tangential evolution.
We seek our reflection like we seek the
water that gives it to us. So be thirsty and
not vain or it will be as if the king with
no clothes started eating himself.

Aoife: How do I become a person?

Dad: Becoming 'someone' is never an easy
thing because you must risk isolation which
is the only true way to 'become'. Many
people cheat by becoming an idea first and
then let the 'someone' grow-up around it
like a weed up a letterbox. The weed is a
mask, the letterbox is who you truly *are*.
Accept a diversity of ideas, do not let the
weed yet. Do not be ideological, instead try

on the hats of your haters, walk in the
shoes of the fanatics, size-up the coat of
the sycophantic and then pull up your socks
and be actively curious, adventurous, and
playfully unaffiliated. In the process let a
person emerge that is a weed free letterbox,
that allows for all types of mail to be
received. Let the letterbox discern, let the
weed die.

Aoife: Would joining a tribe help?

Dad: Socialising is fundamental. However,
people who attach their sense of Self to
ideals are trying to shortcut their Self
development. Joining a tribe means they feel
affiliated. It fools the mind into promoting
Self beyond its obligations. Self is only a
tool, a puppet; do not put it in the
driver's seat. Idealists hand the keys to
Self and then lock who they *really* are in
the boot. They are snowflakes yellow with
the stench of Self and they easily combine
with other unsophisticated Selfs, and then
it snowballs. They might be known as your
'peer', but their growth is different to
yours; it is stilted. In real terms they are
'actors' seeking a scene in which to
'announce' a motivation that leads to
'actor-ing', not action. The snowball size
will determine the extent to which the idea
at the centre of the cooperation is
simplified. The larger the group the simpler
the motivation and the more likely it is to
lead to 'actor-ing', disentanglement and,
ultimately, disintegration. Fundamentally, a
group will oversimplify its motivation if it
becomes too large. 'Actor-ing' is then the
easiest way to express any intent but it is
inconsequential.

Aoife: So, bigger is dumber?

Dad: A defined outcome requires data to be processed; an endeavour that puts a limit on processing will fail. Outcomes must acknowledge rules, lines, and goal posts. Determine your outcome and then let the game begin. Oversimplification will lead to 'fizzling' pieces of unsustainable action. Do not be tribal, instead understand: *Team devotees have a constricted sense of community; they have had their T-shirt tattooed on.* Be an essential cog in the process that can remove itself as the processing changes shape. Consider: *Life is a game, and the ball is not round, so do not place bets.*

Aoife: So, don't be a snowball?

Dad: Be a solitary snowball. It melts and becomes liquid and flows, eddies, erodes, evaporates, wafts and freezes again. It has a dynamic existence filled with phases. Reflect: *The egg came first. Then it became a chicken that would sit on the fence sometimes. The chicken was exposed on the fence but at least it could see the fox, the cat, and the good-intended approach.*

Aoife: Will I be the same as others?

Dad: No one is equal, yet we are all one. There is only one consciousness. In terms of Self, hierarchy is important to survival, but it is a game: *Who has more power, the referee, or the player?*

Aoife: One consciousness?

Dad: Be spiritual. It is recommended. The
terms I use describe my appreciation of
unity, not an abiding belief. The principles
of *oneness* I choose to accept are
universally practiced. In this way, the
terms 'consciousness' and 'awareness' are
functional. I use them accepting that
everyone has a degree of curiosity about
spirit. It is a satisfying curiosity that
can motivate a learning for life. Accept
principles of *oneness* and join me as I
challenge their interpretation. Measure my
spiritual explanations against a logical
dismantling of Self; this is the Self
investigation approach. It is sophistic; it
is not faith.

Aoife: The terms are functional *and*
spiritual?

Dad: For the purpose of this meditation,
consciousness, awareness, Self and mind are
spiritual terms. However, everything is
rendered by the imagination, including
functional notions of unity and separation.
Consequently, I use terms that supposes a
non-dual reality. I am playing with ideas of
unity; the connections I make to science and
other understandings exist to feed
curiosity. Meditation is play, my ideas are
toys, explore them. There are no gurus, be
guided but assume your own journey.

Aoife: Who should I be?

Dad: The 'I' you can never get away from;
the 'observer' you essentially *are*. Let this
be the first truth you accept regardless of
its instability. Self is an avatar emerging

from the mind that is fed by attention.
Attention receives rendered data from the
imagination as it echo-defines everything.
Self builds the connection between a
physical world with limitations and the mind
that cannot experience limitation. The mind
is like a parasite using the hardware of the
body to learn the nature of time and space.
Self manifests in the body as attitude and
habitude. You are meant to be someone who
manipulates their attitude, not someone
who's attitude is to manipulate.

Aoife: I am something I have created?

Dad: 'I' is not created. The *creation* is
your origin-self. 'I' is the 'observer' and
Self is the observed. 'I' is a lens by which
the finite and the infinite are separated.
Self emerges because it is witnessed.

Aoife: What is my origin-self?

Dad: The child you were and *are*. The *child*
is observed and is therefore gifted with
observation; it is innocent and without ego.
This innocence is curiosity; the child is
wise, and the adult is knowledgeable. The
child that is your origin-self is a learner-
for-life; it must explore. Self must allow
for its 'origin' to thrive; the child *is*
eternal inquiry. Your origin-self is the
foundation of Self; it seeks *play* and
occupation. Though it appears to be untrue
for many people, the origin-self is never
forgotten.

Aoife: My *child* Self should be *occupied*?

Dad: Yes, *absorbed* in a task. Recall the child you once were, who would lose hours devoted to a pastime. You were simply completion-focused; it is known as learning. The *child* is integral to an understanding of Self: *not unlike any child, it wants to play and have positive experiences*. The child you *are* loves to travel and yet knows nothing of destinations.

Aoife: Are you my guide?

Dad: My experiences are all I have. I do not know much except what I feel is true. This is not a guidebook it is a meditation. Questions outnumber answers always by one; you are the most interesting person you will ever travel with. However, you can know me; not just as Dad, but as someone inspired by his daughter to inquire. This 'talk', or meditation is one part of your journey. The map has no destination, I will help you draw it.

Aoife: The journey is the destination?

Dad: Yes. So, you have started and arrived at the same time; fundamental consciousness is the reason for the contradiction: *It is infinite; destinations are inconceivable.*

Aoife: Can you explain consciousness?

Dad: There is no language to describe the true nature of awareness. The finite cannot know the infinite. It is a deep calm; it is where you are.

Aoife: What then, is enlightenment?

Dad: A deception, a word with a lost meaning. It once described an intimate appreciation for the true nature of reality.

Aoife: Which is?

Dad: That consciousness is fundamental, and everything is a protrusion from it.

Aoife: How is it achieved?

Dad: It is revealed; it is not achieved. This is the problem with the word 'enlightenment'; it encourages non-enlightenment intentions.

Aoife: What do you mean?

Dad: When 'enlightenment' becomes a pursuit, *something* must be pursued. Consciousness is not a *thing*.

Aoife: How is it revealed?

Dad: In conversation; communication is essential.

Aoife: In conversation with who?

Dad: Your Self.

Aoife: How was it revealed to you?

Dad: I call it mind-blind. The mind 'opens' up into a void and disappears. This *void* is in and composes everything. I have a sense that there are subtle frequency shifts across the 'plane' of this void. For the purposes of Self investigation I call the *shifts* 'protrusions'. In other words, it is close; the distance to it is meaningless. In this way, the process of writing this 'talk' was an awakening.

Aoife: Is reading it a pathway to an awakening?

Dad: There is no path; awareness is available. This 'talk' models an example of Self investigation. In this way it may help you to form your own who-am-I investigation.

Aoife: So, Self investigation is the key?

Dad: It has been my experience. But guidance in ways of investigating is also important. This 'talk' demonstrates a line of questioning consistent with a key understanding.

Aoife: Which is?

Dad: That the inquiry is fulfilment; it is the 'observer'. Therefore, form your questions and never assume you have 'arrived'.

Aoife: Are you a mystic?

Dad: *Everything* is informed by the imagination; do not be deluded. The imagination is pervasive and is a gateway that frames reality. Deep sleep is the exception.

Aoife: Delusion is *not* an act of the imagination?

Dad: Imagination constructs, delusion obstructs. What makes us human is a Self-

awareness that goes beyond Self and
awareness. The mysticism arises as we
attempt to untangle what we truly are from
its representation. In other words, if
seeing the forest *and* the trees
simultaneously is mystical than I am a
mystic. I am not a mystic. I am accidentally
spiritual, and it is ordinary. Our
experience of spirit is ordinary, not
mysterious. It is the feeling we have when
our team wins, our children play, our
friends laugh, our pets snuggle, etc. Spirit
is the extraordinary in the ordinary. My
approach is an invitation to explore the joy
of exploration. It asks you to accept that
accidents are the lessons given as we master
an indirect approach. I am playing with
emerging questions about the true nature of
Self and reality; it is joyous. Laugh with
me.

Aoife: Do I have to go to weddings?

Dad: No. But you will.

Aoife: Can I move things with my mind?

Dad: Yes.

Aoife: How?

Dad: Think — I will move my hand, and your
hand will move.

Aoife: I mean something that is not part of
me.

Dad: Such as?

Aoife: An apple.

Dad: But we are one. The apple is a protrusion from the same plane of consciousness from which you arise. The imagination separates the *thing* 'apple' from the thing you are. Do not let the authorship of the imagination corral your exploration of reality.

Aoife: There are no *things*?

Dad: Defining *things* is an act of Self, *you* are not Self.

Aoife: How do I move the apple?

Dad: Directly.

Aoife: Like my mind 'directly' controlling my hand?

Dad: The mind directly 'informs' the mechanism. You must inform the mechanism that moves apples.

Aoife: Which is?

Dad: Gravity. Anything with mass has gravity. The speed at which you experience time is determined by the distance you are from the source of gravity.

Aoife: So, if I *choose* to leave the apple high in the tree?

Dad: You have made time move faster for the apple with your 'mind'.

Aoife: In other words, I cannot move things with my mind.

Dad: To go *directly* is to travel a distance too short to be meaningful. But it is a step towards infinite possibilities.

Aoife: Am I stupid, or is that explanation confusing?

Dad: Ignorance is the child, it sustains you. Necessarily, some explanations are vague and appear contradictory.

Aoife: Why?

Dad: Removing any objectifiable quality reduces the possibility for Self to hijack the intention. When phrased correctly, explanations of consciousness can be difficult for the imagination to render. Self will then seek other *items* to promote. In meditation you can experience this phenomenon. Close your eyes, bring into your attention the words — myself is known. The *knower* is not defined. Now be keenly aware of the images that come to mind; they are items *promoted* from attention by Self. It is likely that your mind will be momentarily overwhelmed with disassociated data. It leaves most people feeling meditation is 'hard'; the data is distracting. However, the mind is overwhelmed with items because Self is desperately trying to define the *knower*; this is an indication that the meditation is working. Now slow it down — my…Self…is…known. Feel how this interrupts the flow of the data. You may also feel a relaxing of attention. Self is receding.

Aoife: Then my mind is free to move the apple?

Dad: Mind is a consequence of Self. What you are seeking to connect with is like still water, deep and expansive. You are a wave forming on its surface. Self are the bubbles that appear as the water churns. You are a 'protrusion' from the still water. If you wish to break the laws of the physical universe you will have to become *still*.

Aoife: Is that possible?

Dad: Start where you are; understand Self.

Aoife: So, consciousness is infinite?

Dad: Yes. The universe is beauty; it is known by that which knows it as itself. That which *knows* is consciousness and the knowing of the universe as itself is *awareness*. Awareness knows only itself and knows you only as itself; *it* has no other knowledge of any-*thing* including time. From it arises everything, the *everything* is known as processing.

Aoife: Processing?

Dad: Awareness is the 'reason' for processing but has no notion of it. Awareness describes consciousness knowing only itself. It is revealed to us as the 'observer'. The 'observer' *witnesses* the instances that make up time. Time *is* processing. We are processors, like filaments in a radiator expressing heat. We are a necessary expression, allowing for the utility of communication to enable energy dispersion. Our small acts of energy dispersion increase entropy towards all matter 'ripping' apart.

Aoife: Something to look forward to. What happens before that?

Dad: We become one. Electrons? Protons? Neutrons? You are made of them, pick one. Crack it open and count the quarks. Now look for your name on a quark; look very closely. Your initials? Not there? I have quarks too. Oops, we have dropped our quarks; we scramble to recover them. But they have been swapped. It matters not; put your atom back together. Reassemble your molecule and life goes on. Your unique, individual existence shall continue.

Aoife: So, the building blocks of life are in me but are not 'me'.

Dad: Yes.

Aoife: So, what am I?

Dad: You are the *essential* you. *You* are also a collection of old stuff, stuck together in an arrangement that is as necessarily complicated as it needs to be towards increasing entropy. We are a manifestation of everything in the perceived universe that is perfectly imperfect. We must contribute, sustain, explore, manifest all types of processing. In this way communication is fundamental. The dynamic expression of energy consistent with the erupting power of the universe is your mission.

Aoife: Am I an individual?

Dad: The building blocks, fundamental to life, are not individualised; essentially a quark is a quark. Yet their combined arrangement appears to create something individual. It 'appears' to cause individuality. You are not an individual. You are a manifestation of exponential processing, and it is the most beautiful of things. However, your entropic expression, that adds variety to an expanding universe, cannot be replicated; variety is necessary. Your unique activity is also 'captured' on the plane of consciousness in infinitesimally small data points that are, themselves, infinite. In other words, you are writing a unique variation of an eternal theme; make it spectacular.

Aoife: What is entropy?

Dad: For our purposes, it is redundant processing increasing as the size of the non-redundant processing increases. Variation in the universe must also increase.

Aoife: Is variation the same as entropy?

Dad: No. The universe may be an eternally opening flower. Each movement reveals new details; the kinetics appears to bring forth change. In this way variation might be endless; there may be no ultimate ripping-apart of everything. However, I tend to accept an entropic interpretation that allows for variation to increase.

Aoife: How do I erupt with the power of the universe?

Dad: Communicate. All processes have properties, and all communication is a process. Revelation brought about by the intersection of words and ideas promotes renewal. In this way, 'words' are like agents of processing. 'Actions' may speak louder than words, but words do have kinetic potential. Words act like atoms, they form thought-molecules that become idea-stuff, that are then itemised in attention. Atoms are not defined by clear boundaries; their periphery is a point at which energy fades and words are much the same. Listening then becomes a fundamental process in an expanding universe. It is an *expansion* of understanding that relies on engagement. In this way engagement *is* awareness: *Awareness is a lens, engagement is an iris, 'made' of consciousness.* Effective listening is the first step towards bringing-forth the 'power' of the infinite.

Aoife: How can consciousness know 'only' itself.

Dad: Imagine there is a 'bump' on the plane of consciousness. This bump is *made* of consciousness; known to itself as itself. This 'protrusion' is populated with many other protrusions, which are populated with many other protrusions, etc such as we are: *We are an entropic 'protrusion' from the plane of consciousness.* Consciousness is not divided, it is one; we are one.

Aoife: So, consciousness is me and us but knows only itself?

Dad: It may help to imagine consciousness as an alien, without form or time, using your

'awareness' as a portal to observe the
focused state it assumes, that is your mind.
You might like to imagine the alien is
'amazed' by the limitations the human mind
places on it. Imagine its normal state is
without memory, muscles, thoughts, actions,
emotion, hair, fingernails, eyeballs, etc.
One day this alien will park the hardware of
your body and mind in the garage of the
physical universe and exit. It will then
return to its massless, timeless state; like
the relaxing of it that occurs during deep
sleep. Memory, sensation, dreams, dimension,
and purpose will cease to exist; essentially
all the appearances of time, that we define
as our 'being', will end. We know it as
death. Further to this imagine the 'alien'
is enveloped in a membrane, like a hazmat
suit. Inside the membrane there is no time,
outside is our universe. The 18 Billion
years or so that it will take for our
universe to disperse all its kinetic
potential would appear instantaneous to the
alien. Or more accurately, it would be an
'instant', composed *of* the alien.

Aoife: But there is no 'alien'.

Dad: We are a protrusion arising from the
plane of consciousness. This protrusion is
like a bump printed on a page of braille.
Except the page is consciousness and knows
only itself: *Imagine the bump is without
mass; it can only be known to consciousness
as itself.* So then imagine that fundamental
massless particles act like conduits
piercing the membrane separating the finite
and the infinite. But remember consciousness
knows only itself and the protrusion, that
you are, is known by consciousness as

itself. Consciousness is infinite and therefore has no notion of the Big Bang; consciousness cannot know time.

Aoife: But *everything* is a protrusion from consciousness including time?

Dad: Yes, and it is known to it as itself. The 18 billion years, or so, it will take for our universe to cool will not be 'visible' to the plane of consciousness even though it is known to it. Consciousness is not intelligent. The gift of intelligence is given to the finite informed by time and space, or in relative terms, mind and body. The finite cannot know the infinite and the infinite has no experience; yet from the infinite comes the building blocks of your perceived existence. In this way, the 'building blocks' are the conduit.

Aoife: Forest for the trees?

Dad: And trees for the forest. X-rays 'see' bone but not skin, but we see skin and not the bone. It is impossible for the naked eye to 'see' X-rays but we perceive their existence evidentially. Evidentially we perceive the 'building blocks' as the 'observer' concealed behind Self. The 'observer' is a focusing of consciousness and purveys processing; exclusively. The 'observer' can *only* see processing. During deep sleep, the 'observer' relaxes back-into pure consciousness.

Aoife: The universe is a process?

Dad: Yes. It is an answer to the question 'why is there something rather than

nothing?', or more specifically, 'why should
there be a protrusion from the plane of
consciousness?' But from the point of view
of process ontology this question is
senseless. Processing is the expression of
all available processing that expresses all
available energy types to enable continuous
cycles of processing that increase entropy
etc and it matters not when it started or
how: *Processing will forever be the only
consequence of processing.* Therefore, the
Big Bang can be regarded as a process-start-
up that is an *answer* to the question. Or,
more specifically, is an answer to a
slightly different question - why is there
something where there should be nothing?
Therefore, the entire chaos and apparent
separation of everything in the universe is
an entropic act towards equilibrium. The
resulting consequence of which allows for
the expansion and subsequent ripping apart
of everything.

Aoife: So, the universe is consciousness
answering the question, 'should there be
some-*thing?*' with, No!

Dad: The universe is an engine in slow decay
driven to disperse energy: *A return to near
nothingness is the answer.*

Aoife: Am I 'something'?

Dad: There is a massive amount of energy to
be processed as the universe cools. Like a
volcanic flow hitting the cool ocean waters,
the rock does not instantly solidify. Small
cascades of flow keep populating and will do
so until all useful and redundant energy is

expressed. You are a cascade adding variety to an eternal cooling.

Aoife: I am a *cascade*?

Dad: If we accept the universe is a cooling process and is the answer to the question — why is there something when there should be nothing? We can begin to accept our role: *We are irradiators helping the cooling by dispersing heat as we add variation.* Accept your role as an exquisite expression of variation. The more active you are the more heat you help disperse. When you express your use of energy with vigour and a sense of unity you are entirely consistent with the function of the universe. It is then that you will feel a powerful sense of purpose. You will also feel incredible satisfaction. It will afford you a sense of the infinite which is spirituality. It will also mean that Self will not force questions such as — what is the purpose of life?

Aoife: What is the purpose of life?

Dad: The purpose of life is to arrive at a state of awareness that means Self will never *know* the need to ask - what is the purpose of life? In this way, the purpose is to be entropic. There are no obstacles to the fulfilment of your happiness. There is activity that is redundant, there is activity that is useful, and then there is the by-product; it is *available* information. In other words, we take the good and the bad because of the rest. The bad manifests in the good to create the opportunity for further manifestations; the purpose of life is to be the something that comes from nothing. In this way, happiness is the appreciation of the closeness of everything. Therefore, appreciate the space *between,* because any objective pursuit of happiness is an act of Self. Self can never be happy, and you are not Self.

Aoife: Is Self a 'what' or a 'who'?

Dad: Self is not you. Or, in the terms of your question, Self is a 'what' that believes it is a 'who' and it is not 'what' you essentially are. It finds its origin in consciousness.

Aoife: Will time always exist?

Dad: Perceive time as a mistake. Time is as close to a perfect perception-error as is possible. So close to perfect that it may never have been perceived. But it is and its imperfection is the reason for its persistence. However, time is best understood as instantaneous infinities being created towards the end of all kinetic activity. Fundamentally time does not exist; entropy 'exists' and we 'experience' it as time. If you imagine entropy as an algorithm built upon simple 'laws' time would not be represented. Time would be the gap between the algorithmic elements; time is the 'feeling' we have when reading a piece of data that compels us to read the next piece of the algorithm and so on. *2+2=4* time is the 'momentum' that exists between the stimuli '2' and '+' etc.

Aoife: So, time will end?

Dad: So long as there is kinetics the cooling of the universe will continue: *Kinetic energy, however, will eventually dissipate; entropically.* Time is, possibly, a helictical looping of expanding space stuff. This looping will lose momentum ultimately and everything will end very suddenly; or so it shall appear. But essentially time does not exist. There is only ever 'now'. This is not easy to perceive but let us accept that if time stopped so too would a particle zooming around the nucleus of an Atom. However, this particle is also a wave and to 'see' the wave time must restart. If you 'pause' a wave there is nothing to 'see'. So, time is a 'witness' of entropy. Or more accurately, time is a lens that allows for consciousness to be focused, moment by moment. The content of a moment will not tolerate substantiation, and this is entropy.

Aoife: Is time in my head?

Dad: Time can be understood as a construct of the mind; that exists in a timeless and time respondent state simultaneously. In this way, the *mind* is composed of consciousness, which composes everything. Time is now, now is an instant, an instant is incomparable; it is meaningless. Likewise, the more we retreat into the image of Self beyond its origin the less it seems to change with time.

Aoife: So, is time a collection of *nows*?

Dad: Think of time as the populating of infinitesimally small 'data-points' on the plane of consciousness. Each moment is 'documented' on this plane as an *instant*. It is the stringing together of these 'instances' that creates a *sense* of time.

Aoife: Like a movie?

Dad: Maybe. Look closely at an instant and the one next to it; they are separated by a distance that is meaningless. The act of comparing two concurrent instances is equivalent to dividing *now*. This is at the centre of the idea that in any given instant everything is as it should be. Reflect: *In an instant nothing can be substantiated.* Any attempt to substantiate or justify the content of any instant will fail.

Aoife: Without time, we are substance-*less*.

Dad: Yes.

Aoife: When will I be my *forever* Self?

Dad: You are writing your own story. Your life is a story your mind tells itself. Letting the authorship of the mind limit who you will become is a mistake I hope I can help you avoid. Understanding that Self has an origin - the origin-self, and its ability to be described as childlike has significance. Those who accept an inner-child concept of Self often do so because the image of a 'child' comes easily to mind regarding Self. Given, that much of what happens in the mature mind is concerned with the creation of a story that the mind tells itself towards enabling a character called personality playing roles in society which is purely an expression of entropy, it is strange that the origin-self has the feeling

that it is separate to the mind-creating-
mind story. It is almost as if the origin-
self is a mysterious inspiration that helps
the Self story to begin. It is not, the
origin-self is the foundation storyteller
from which *mind* and *Self* emerge
simultaneously. This is subsequent to the
rendering performed by the imagination. It
is for this reason that Self is understood
to be significantly shaped early in life.

Aoife: How do I shape it?

Dad: Your story is heavily informed by the
processing that is the cooling of the
universe. The expression of your eternal
qualities must be consistent with the
activity of the universe. Your activity is
an opportunity for energy to move through
processes entropically. The massive cooling
event that is the expansion of the universe
is a process that must be mostly
destructive, again towards entropy.
Destruction in the universe does not mean
destroyed. Your experience should be a
constant cycle of reconfiguring. This
process should involve the destruction of
most constructs towards almost complete
annihilation. Let the seed of functionality
that remains enliven new constructs. If it
were not in our nature to evolve in this
one-step-forward-99.99%-of-a-step-back
manner we would be two-year-old throwing
tantrums forever. Consider: *Tantrum is a
process, intended mostly for the release of
energy. The small nugget of functionality it
informs includes the acquisition of a more
sophisticated communication style. It
encourages a refocusing of purpose and this
increases the complexity of the human*

31

'system'. Remember: *The tantrum itself has low entropy. The negotiation, politeness, conciliation, and concessions learnt because of it are a more diverse expression of energy; they are entropic.*

Aoife: Entropy is important to you?

Dad: Regard processes that increase entropy as being 'in-tune' with the expanding nature of the universe. In this way, processing should be an expression of many energy 'types'. Communication is at the centre of this. Imagine all communication types – the News Anchor coordinating with the teleprompter, the surgeon communicating with the scapple, the landscaper interacting with the earth, the mother singing to her baby, the sperm communing with the egg. There is nothing more diverse in the human experience than communication. It is the central enabling element of all endeavours, and you are managing a unique section of its spectrum. Now imagine communication as a transferal of energy. Including energy wasted, conserved and utilised. Now consider the number of communication types you are committed to. Consider all aspects of communication – the conversation with a loved one and the textual and kinaesthetic conversation you have with a knife as you apply the peanut butter. Your spectrum of communication commitments is diverse and pervasive. The universe expands because of the communitive cascading of energy; they are correlations. Humans are a demonstration of energy consumption based on the same principle; we are not separate from the fundamental mechanisms of the universe. Processes that involve an awareness of many communication styles will be excited towards enabling Self development.

Aoife: So Self awareness is the goal?

Dad: It is important. In a process focused ontological understanding *revelation* is central: Self is a *construct*; its demotion *reveals* awareness. The idea then is to experience life's journey as the destination separate from Self. Self masks the essential you, the 'protrusion' promoted from consciousness that you *truly* are. Essentially, Self is something you have created, or more accurately, the mind has created so it can place a character into the story it tells itself. The creation of a Self is the first 'in-tune' process you initiate. By 'in-tune' I mean it is consistent with entropy: *Self is an ordering of socially enabling agents. Its creation causes destruction and construction in almost equal measure. The small part of it that is not destroyed exist to enable more processing towards the expiration of energy. This is understood by accepting that the larger the universe becomes the more disordered it is. The purpose of the disorder is to use energy and create new opportunities to create platforms for the use of more energy. Therefore, nearly all activity is destructive. 'Destructive' in this sense is best understood as renewal. For example, the energy that is the consequence of creating Self will be expressed socially.* 'Self awareness' allows for Self to be seen for what it is.

Aoife: And what is it?

Dad: Self exists to help ensure your genes
will be passed on; an ultimate act of
communication or 'processing'. Its other key
function is to make sure the next generation
creates a Self that is also socially viable.
Consider: *If we were Mudworms our succession
would be our business. But we are social
beings and therefore we need a Self.* Self is
a tool, a very persistent and present tool,
designed to make us socially viable.
Specifically, it is a collection of tools
consisting of anger, conciliation, courtesy,
forgiveness, joy, love etc. The process of
creating this collection of tools is arduous
and requires lesson being learnt mostly the
hard way. Self helps you mitigate and
reconcile the forces of *want* and *need.* This
lesson is painfully learnt by a two-year-old
throwing a tantrum in the supermarket; the
parent is embarrassed but so too is the
child: *It attracts the wrong type of
attention, inconsistent with social
viability.*

Aoife: So 'I' am not Self?

Dad: 'I' is not Self, yet Self comes from
'I'. Imagine you are a carpenter with a tool
belt full of many different types of
communication tools, collectively they are
Self. Some tools are chosen impulsively,
others discerningly. Now consider who is the
'who' choosing the tool — the carpenter? The
'carpenter' is the 'I' that you are when you
are not your *tools.*

Aoife: So, 'I' uses Self but 'I' is not
Self?

Dad: 'I' *observes* Self and Self is not *you.*
However, it can appear to be all *you* are.
Fundamentally, many people believe they *are*
their reactions, feelings and thoughts.
However, regard these as components of Self
as *observed* by 'I'.

Aoife: So, Self is a display?

Dad: Yes. Identify feelings such as anger
and love as an 'act' of Self. In development
Self accumulates processes for managing the
protection of the physical *being* you are
towards social viability. Imagine, Self is a
processor; it is entropic. In this way a
healthy Self processes data cyclically. Self
is a tool, like a compass, to give you a
heading towards your next acquisition of
tools. Self is inquiring like a compass is
guiding.

Aoife: How do you perceive your own Self?

Dad: I have always had a sense of my Self as
a separate entity. I 'view' my Self outside
of my body.

Aoife: Can I do that?

Dad: Yes. We all do it. It is my belief that
Self is developed from an out-of-body
perspective. I believe a child is inclined,
in a trial-and-error manner, to view
themselves remotely. This helps them echo-
define their environment; enabled by the
imagination. Self is a construct of the mind
informed by time and space. It is,
therefore, entirely logical that we would
become more reliant on Self as it becomes
more stable; it is a dynamic expression of

survival. It is also how we help increase
entropy. Consequently, early in life we
'forget' how to view ourselves remotely.
This also makes the visualising of your
origin-self as a *child* logical. The
development of Self required you to view the
child you were remotely; that 'perspective'
will, therefore, be the view point you adopt
of Self as you age. Consequentially,
awareness is described as an eternal
'observer'. Arguably, this is our default,
pre *Self* state: *Conceptualise an infant as
infinity 'assimilating' with a manifestation
of itself informed by entropy.* The
development of the Self tools is a logical
progression.

Aoife: Why is it significant?

Dad: Remember our objective is to express
energy as dynamically as possible towards
increasing entropy. The most powerful
example of this is procreation: *With every
human life created entropy increases.*
Additionally, working towards an
understanding of infinity as a 'plane' from
which we are all a 'protrusion' — known to
us as consciousness, is, like the creation
of life itself, an elemental expression of
energy. The questions 'where do we come
from? Why are we here?' appear to be as old
as time itself. We have been looking to the
sky for answers forever. To help entropy
increase we must expand into the heavens.
Therefore, we must have more people, more
activity, more questions and *every* possible
perspective must find a vantage point.
Fundamentally, like the didgeridoo player
breathing in and out at the same time, Self

must be observed and embodied
simultaneously.

Aoife: Why do we *lose* the 'remote'
perspective?

Dad: We appear to 'lose' the ability to view
ourselves remotely early in life because
Self becomes our main operating system. The
'predominance' of Self is essential to help
increase entropy. However, we can easily
become *too much* Self. Ego then becomes a
problem.

Aoife: How?

Dad: Ego has no connection to consciousness
and is necessarily Self involved; it must
ensure the survival of the being.

Aoife: So, Self limits our perspective?

Dad: Yes. We do not 'lose' the ability to
view ourselves objectively, we 'push' it
aside. Or, more precisely, it becomes
obscured by Self. For everyone, at some
point in life, the question will present
itself — how can my life have more meaning?
This is the 'observer' you essentially are,
telling you it is time to engage in an
elemental aspect of existence. In other
words, the 'question' is telling you it is
time for you to be energised by infinity.
You will probably start with *reimaging* your
origin-self, and 'seeing' if they are
reconciled. In this way, you *become* the
'observer'; it is the awareness
'perspective'. You can then begin to
interact with Self with a sense of distance.

Aoife: How do I *reimagine* my origin-self?

Dad: Look at it. Reimagined does not mean reconstructed. The child is *you*. Literally, it is the image you have of yourself as a child; it cannot be destroyed. It must be acknowledged as a *living* aspect of your Self; the catalyst of it. In this way, it can be given new intentions, occupations and means of inquiry. See the child and ask - are you absorbed? The origin-self or inner-child is like any child, they want to *do* something. Give them a brush to paint with, give them a needle to sew with, give them some clay to mould, give them a song to sing, give them blocks to build with, give them a pen to write with. Remember a time when you were 'absorbed' in tasks with no notion of the wider world, or Self. This child is still you and it is actively informing the choices Self makes — give it back its interests, wonder, craft. Simple? Yes. But unfortunately, *conditions* of Self such as fear of judgement, fear of failure, fear of missing your favourite TV show, fear generally means most people would rather not 'look' for it, and subsequently they *neglect,* their origin-self. They let the child they *are* sit in the dark corner of their attention disenchanted. This is the first mistake many make towards awareness; Self must not be discarded. Entropy must increase, any simple act of creation is consistent with that inevitability. If your inner-child loved colouring in, then help entropy increase, pick up some pencils, find some designs, express some redundant energy and give your life some colour.

Aoife: What does your Self *feel* like to you?

Dad: I am driving a body by adopting a point-of-view position. I have a sense that this body has limits. I imagine consciousness 'pushing' me towards processing. I accept that 'mind' is a process *author*. I realise that the path of least resistance is not straight and available resources are often more plentiful than they first appear. Essentially, I am a puppet master controlling a body that will die; when 'I' let go of the strings time will end and a massless freedom will persist.

Aoife: Puppet master?

Dad: We are either controlled by the puppet or we are the puppet master. My approach attempts to put you in control of Self. However, for the most part, the people you encounter will be slaves to the puppet.

Aoife: What about death?

Dad: Once the strings are released all memory, attention, feeling or sense of Self dissolves; an unknowable deep calm emerges.

Aoife: Unknowable?

Dad: The 'knowing' of things is a condition of Self. In other words, knowing is over-rated. The realising of your true nature is an uncoded, deidentified state that removes any sense that you are limited by individuality. Individuality is also a 'condition' of Self; an important construct for social 'beings'. But if you meditate and can conceive an absolute, 'Universal'

freedom, individuality begins to feel like
an imposition or a necessary shackling to
processing. True joy never is and never will
be associated with Self.

Aoife: That reminds me, *ego must ensure the
survival of the being,* so ego is good?

Dad: Yes. But it must 'express' its
objective; it can become *toxic.* Imagine ego
is the captain of a ship with the sole
purpose to navigate a community towards
fulfilment. Or in other words, to make
babies and give them confidence. If, for
example, ego is used to make money for its
own sake or used to develop a persona that
does not enable others, then it will create
ill-defined feelings of deficiency. Often
this deficiency will be compensated for with
acts of Self centred gratification, often
harmful because of the necessary
anesthetising. Ego 'relaxes' once it 'sees'
that it is *powering* a Self that has
something more important to care for than
itself, such as a child: *This does not mean,
however, everyone must literally 'have a
baby'.* Increasing entropy requires the
expansion of community – do something for
the expansion.

Aoife: I feel like a 'decentralised' ego
will compromise my sense of identity?

Dad: Ego is not 'central'. It is more like a
network of energy; the more you enable its
outreach potential the more empowering it
becomes. The question really is, what is
your identity without ego? Or, if we are all
protrusions from the 'same' plane of
consciousness then, without ego, will we all

be the same? Do we risk becoming the same kind of enlightened-zombie? Good question, and as you begin to become aware, or more accurately, as you become to acknowledge that you *are* awareness, questions like this seem valid. Reflect: *Driftwood attract crustaceans, seaweeds and other 'protrusions'. Do not look at the barnacles on the encrusted driftwood and think you are seeing the timber. Look through the protrusions and see the wood. The 'barnacles' that make up you consist of Self tools. Now imagine they are more like filters that help separate the infinite world of the wood and the finite world of the 'protrusions'.* Consciousness looks *into* the finite world through the senses of the protrusion; through the unique lens created by your unique Self filters.

Aoife: Self makes my 'colour' on the spectrum of communication unique?

Dad: Yes.

Aoife: So, I am not just a processor in the entropy generator known as the universe?

Dad: Process focused ontology is not bleak. It might be unfamiliar but, essentially, it is an invitation to sense an expansive freedom. We are craft-creatures. Everything about our entropic responsibilities is enabled by inquiry. Your inquisitions must have redundancies and tangents. Accept that we are each responsible for the refinement of communication. We are invited to craft communication towards a never ending enabling of community.

Aoife: What is a craftsperson?

Dad: An explorer of the *way* things are done.
Imagine you are an adventurer, hungry for
the adventure *with no interest in
destinations.* Then imagine the adventurer
you are is a character in a game, their
perceptions, interactions, and thoughts are
the ingredients of the character's Self.
Hopefully, these ingredients are well
developed for the purpose of social
viability. The game is a manifestation or
expression of entropy so regard all that is
'matter' or 'real' in the game as ultimately
reducible to something massless. Now close
your eyes, put down the controller that is
Self. More accurately, imagine your entire
body is the controller and step back from
it. Gain a sense of the 'observer' that is
the *true* you. It has always been there,
aware only of itself. It needs only itself
and will know only itself and nothing else;
it will not know time or memory or body or
mind. It is the plane of consciousness from
which we protrude. It is a 'shared' plane;
we are one. The 'stuff' of the physical
world is a layering of illusionary elements.

Aoife: The physical world does not exist?

Dad: It is illusion-*ary.* Remember: *Don't
look at the barnacles on the encrusted
driftwood and think you are seeing the
timber. Look through the barnacles and see
the wood. Now imagine the wood is timeless,
infinite and the growths and barnacles are
components of the 'perceived' physical world
'protruding' from the driftwood.* The
protrusions do not indicate the 'true'

origin or state of things; they are
illusionary.

Aoife: But it all looks 'real'?

Dad: As it should. Time is the reason why we
perceive things as substantive. Without time
there is no 'substance'; there can be no
place without time, there can be no time
without place. It is like a computer trying
to understand the electricity that runs it.
It might try to stop the flow of electricity
momentarily to investigate it. But then the
electricity appears to no longer 'exist' and
the computer no longer has the *power* to
investigate anything. Now imagine the
componentry of the computer, and the keys,
the screen, etc. are also 'made' of
electricity. Now when the computer tries to
stop the flow not only will it lose power,
but the computer itself will also, literally
cease to exist. Consequently, the questions
raised by consciousness are *hard*. Once
again, the finite cannot know the infinite
and the infinite knows only itself and
'knows' the finite *only* as itself.

Aoife: So then, consciousness *is* fundamental
in the universe?

Dad: However, a fundamental theory of
consciousness is *only* a theory. Which
fortunately, grants you the opportunity to
hypothesise and to consider: *There is no
separation between things.* It also allows
you to look at '1' and '0' and think - from
simple things grows inconceivable
complexity. It enables analogies: *Imagine
ice being aware of itself as a cube with no
knowledge of other water states. Now imagine*

*it trying to make sense of the liquid water
it sits in and is 'made' of; imagine the
water is timeless and limitless. The
dispersed, endless nature of the 'liquid'
would be impossible for the cube to
conceive. The cube would only have the sense
that it was floating somehow.* Like the ice,
we are confined by time and space, but we
can 'sense' that we are floating in a
'medium' of which we appear to be 'made';
meditation helps.

Aoife: Is it then a theory for theory's
sake?

Dad: The 'feeling' of consciousness presents
a genuine *hard* problem scientifically. The
'experience' of consciousness cannot *yet* be
explained by simply identifying brain
activity. Therefore, a gap exists, and many
people, like me, try to bridge the gap by
describing the 'pervasiveness' of
consciousness. Science must find the answer
to this *hard* problem. I provide qualitative
data that responds to an intuitive
hypothesis; it is scientifically
insignificant. Except that, all predictions
are the grandchildren of experience and
intuition. The pursuit of an answer should
lead to more questions in an endless cycle
towards entropy; this is fundamental.
Increasingly, the cycling will become less
objective; this is also fundamental.
Subsequently, Self will recede.

Aoife: Will consciousness ever be
understood?

Dad: We are unable to conceive the true
nature of consciousness; consciousness is

infinite. We can *sense* the eternal nature of it through meditation and awakening. But it is entirely impossible for an entity existing in time and space to experience infinity. Therefore, the only purpose of discovery is to create new opportunities of discovery; in this way it is already understood. This eternal cycle-of-inquiry is as close as we can hope to be to a sense of infinity and that is why the purpose of life is to process. Consider: *'Something' exists because of entropy. The light turns off and the globe cools; the universe is the cooling after the light has gone out.* The Big Bang is like an incandescent globe that burns brightest just before the element breaks. The Big Bang was not the start of something it was an ending; a slow, complicated dispersion and correlation of energy towards the cooling of everything.

Aoife: What is the purpose of imagination?

Dad: Our imagination is echo-defining your experience, helping your mind tell itself a story. Imagine consciousness is a type of reflective plane containing bits of data informed by a one-step-forward-99.99%-of-a-step-back process.

Aoife: one-step-forward-99.99%-of-a-step-back?

Dad: Yes. Stand up and step it out. The pattern created, essentially, is a type of oscillation, or vibration. It is a pattern that allows for the 'mapping' of everything and the creation of correlations.

Aoife: The imagination vibrates?

Dad: Everything vibrates. The imagination
echo-defines everything vibrationally,
everything that appears in your sensors,
real or not real.

Aoife: Real or not real?

Dad: The image of an apple in your minds-eye
is rendered by the imagination and is placed
into attention. It is then equally
substantive in attention as a *real* apple.
This is the reason why doubt, insecurity and
other *imagined* conditions of Self conjure
strident responses. The imagination *makes*
them substantive. However, doubt and
insecurity, etc are *always* present and are
constantly being rendered and placed into
attention along with all other 'items'
defined by the sensors. Doubt, insecurity,
loneliness, anger, etc will only become part
of the story the mind is writing if Self
puts it there. Self 'promotes' these 'items'
in attention because it learnt to associate
them with maintaining your social viability.

Aoife: Why *items*?

Dad: Remember, the imagination renders
everything, making all real and unreal data
substantive, or in other words, making them
into 'items'. For the mind to write the
story it tells itself in needs all promoted
data to be substantive. Imagine the mind is
hanging trinkets on a bracelet chain, it
cannot hang the 'idea' of something; it
hangs rendered items. It is the reason why
when, doubt, loneliness, anger etc, are
promoted by Self associated images or
experiences arise. Very often our 'feelings'

are preceded by a memory that consists of textual data — images or sensations. These *unreal* items appear *real* in the mind.

Aoife: Because the imagination 'rendered' them?

Dad: Yes.

Aoife: Tell me again, where do I find enlightenment?

Dad: Remember consciousness, fundamental to the universe, is revealed and is not a place you arrive at. It is always present.

Aoife: Will I know it when I see it?

Dad: It is not mystical. It is not monumental or magical. In many ways, it is about the absence of things. It is not essential for a definition of enlightenment to associate with mysticism. It simply means, a state of understanding. It is not a *way* of understanding; it is not a *state* of mind. Reflect: *Activate your sense of fundamentality.*

Aoife: And in many ways it is about the absence of - what?

Dad: Self. I define Self as a collection of characteristics that make up your personality. Your personality is the socially enabling version of Self 'observed' by *you*. Towards *enlightenment* I use the term 'observer'. The 'observer' is you as a *realised* consciousness. The 'observer' is not intelligent beyond social contexts. Children learn to develop Self from the 'observer' perspective. However, with the assertion of Self, or in other words, when we cease Self inquiry, we blindfold the 'observer'. I am asking you to re-acquire this third-person perspective, reenergise your Self inquiry. However, it can only teach you something in a social setting; this is a great power.

Aoife: How do I know if my Self is *viable*?

Dad: The cycles of processing it activates should be short and enabling or oscillating. In other words, the 'tools' of Self are inadequate when the arch of an issue or problem never assumes a waveform. If we regard awareness as the axis around which cycles of your Self loop, the wave form created should be balanced. The peak of a wave might be a revelation which then subsides towards a contemplative mind-set prompting more questions, that lead down towards confusion and challenge before rising again motivated by the power of inquiry. If the peak does not subside and the trough does not rise again then Self is socially inadequate. The excessive use of anger, for example, means for Self's anger dimension the waveform is shapeless. Anger is a generic response, which is Self in protection mode. Anger is the most dynamic way to restart stalled processes: *It is an indicator that a Self has limited processing options. It is also a warning to others.*

Aoife: What is meditation?

Dad: Meditation is a means for attaining a state of being that *recognises* the infinite. The greatest expanse you are ever likely to

conceive, all the greatest sense of space
you are possibly able to sense is not the
heavens above. A true sense of the infinite
comes about because of 'mindlessness'
achieved through meditation. Meditation
needs practice but doesn't necessarily
require time. Meditation is less about a
comfortable sitting position and incense and
is more about your readiness to 'give-way'
to consciousness.

Aoife: Is my life predetermined?

Dad: Everything is consciousness.
Consciousness may be described as an endless
plane of data-points that 'captures'
information known as instances. You help
'create' those data points with observations
made from your unique perspective, but they
are consciousness; we all inform the same
'point' in time and space but from different
perspectives. Awareness allows us to *sense*
those data points without the limitations of
time and space. We can't *be* consciousness
because it is infinite but, vibrationally we
can be energised by its limitless nature.
This is characterised by an awareness of
oneness, and this may be the reason why some
people feel a strong sense of destiny.
Remember: *We are not one with everything,
everything is one.*

Aoife: So, nothing is determined?

Dad: The deterministic view may be
understood if we accept that consciousness
will be expressed in us towards the
manifestation of a process. Any act that
allows for this kind of *flow* may feel
connected to a bigger concept that is beyond

manipulation. Relatively, we are brutish beasts of burden; we are built to process. Your life is scripted in so far as it is determined you *will* process data with the utility of communication, including redundant and *residual* communication types. Imagine the vibratory nature of the *expression-of-consciousness* you essentially are is an expression of energy types. This includes redundant and residual energy. It is therefore *determined* that all processing produces the same vibratory expression of energy.

Aoife: What *is* communication?

Dad: It is best understood as the correlations in a process. Words are systems, they change and respond to their environment, or *context*. The interaction of two words inevitably, increases the complexity of meaning and interpretation: *Allowing for tangents and randomness to emerge, sometimes redundantly.* This is the definition of entropy. Remember: *Entropy must increase, this is fundamental - communication must 'increase'.* Communication is interaction, interaction is correlation, correlations create randomness, randomness includes redundant qualities, redundancies must increase and so communication is fundamental. Put two words together - congratulations, you have just increased entropy, or behaved in a manner consistent with the fundamental nature of the universe.

Aoife: How then, should I communicate with people?

Dad: As the 'observer'. Do not talk to others as Self. Self is a set of personality qualities like the dressing in the window of a shop. Use Self as a profile, advertising your social viability. The Self part of you, essentially is the part of the iceberg that you see above the water. Consider: *The larger part of the iceberg, unseen beneath the surface, brings the part above into existence. Above the surface is Self, below is awareness; it is from where our 'authenticity' emerges.* Self 'announces' your social intent; once an initial presentation is made to others be prepared to 'bring-forth' the *'observer'* you truly are. Remember: the 'observer' is consciousness. In meditation, practice your ability to 'conjure' the 'observer'. I suggest you create an image of yourself as playfully unaffiliated and a journey focused adventurer. These two dimensions personify consciousness manifesting in you as the 'observer' and can be a means of 'initiating' awareness. Remember: *consciousness should be regarded as a network of infinitesimally small data points permeating all time and space; memory is made of these 'points'. Your 'conscious' interaction with others informs these points.*

Aoife: So, I shouldn't be my-*Self*?

Dad: Be *authentic*. It is important to acknowledge - Self will compensate for, mimic and obscure consciousness; Self will *override*. Imagine Self is an actor — it does not need to 'consider' anything, but it knows how to 'recite' indicative phrases. It must be put aside otherwise you risk

interacting with people as if you are
waiting to for your 'turn' to talk and that
is 'acting'; instead listen and be
reflective. Subsequently consciousness is
not an actor and will not 'recite'; it is
absorbing *your* environment. If consciousness
is 'present' you might feel that your recall
is working instinctively and you have an
effortless ability to visualise:
Consciousness is 'using' your mind as a
'visualising' tool, to 'see' what you see.
If allowed consciousness will look through
your 'Self (the actor) as if it were a
series of filters. If the curtain is pulled
back consciousness will see through the
window *made* of Self and project-out who you
truly are. In this analogy consciousness is
literally the 'observer'. The curtain is
ego, pull it back by understanding the
purpose of ego.

Aoife: So, memory is important to
authenticity?

Dad: It is an indicator that you are *aware*
in the moment. Memory is activated by
awareness. If you also accept that
consciousness is fundamental in the universe
and is, essentially, a set of
infinitesimally small data points, then
imagine these points 'trap' data. These
traps 'absorb' every instant creating the
illusion of time. These consciousness 'data-
points' become 'available' to us during
times of low intensity processing: *Deep*
sleep, for instance, is a 'falling' into
pure awareness, but is also a time for
memory consolidation. Accept then, that this
data *is* memory and is available because of
awareness. Awareness is consciousness as the

'observer', it is consciousness as experienced within 'time'.

Aoife: Awareness is the creator, looking 'through' the creation as it creates its own past?

Dad: Yes. But it 'sees' the creation only as itself; it does not literally create anything. Remember: *Memories are items that can be promoted in attention; they are objectifiable.* The imagination echo-defines your environment to provide data to the mind so it can tell a story to itself. Emotional reactions to items promoted in attention *are* the story the mind is telling that then exist to inform the next chapter. Awareness is *available* to the mind as the mind continues to inform Self or, in other words, continues to shape the character featured in its story.

Aoife: So, it is through the mind that I inform Self with awareness; and its availability to 'all' data?

Dad: It is the mind that 'receives' awareness, and awareness *is* available. This data is *known* to the mind as something Self has promoted. The mind *knows* no difference between the *available* nature of awareness, and something promoted by Self.

Aoife: How do I identify authenticity?

Dad: Learn to recognise when you are speaking to a *Self* and not the 'observer'. Self-*dependant* people are not effective listeners. Some learn to 'act' as listener; they are replicating authenticity based on a notion they have of the 'observer'. However, these types of 'actors' are not good at *growing* conversation. They cannot follow tangents they do not own.

Aoife: What do I do?

Dad: You can 'model' the 'observer' for others. In this way acknowledge that Self has weaknesses. Self does not like ignorance, Self likes to 'know' things. Therefore, adopt a playfully unaffiliated persona; your-Self will struggle to dominate: *Authentic learners are not Self-orientated.*

Aoife: But Self likes to know things?

Dad: There is a difference between knowing and learning. Self gets bored, learners get task orientated. boredom is Self questioning the social viability of a lesson given in the *now*. Learning is addiction to astonishment; it is inquiry that leads to further inquiry, consistent with the fundamental nature of the universe.

Aoife: Is astonishment a reflection of authenticity?

Dad: Yes. Do not seek to have your viewpoints substantiated or to have your opinion validated; listen for and reflect authenticity. Invite the 'observer' in others to 'push' their Self aside.

Aoife: What then is *reflected* back to me when I look in the mirror?

Dad: Something the imagination has rendered.

Aoife: I am rendered?

Dad: Self is rendered.

Aoife: Self sees the character it is?

Dad: The character the mind has created. You are looking at a puppet.

Aoife: But it looks real?

Dad: There is a difference between illusionary and illusion. Essentially, the imagination is making the puppet substantive, it does not make alterations to its *form*. The imagination is responsible for separating the world into items. Looking into a mirror is powerfully substantive; Self is instantly assured as to the stability of its existence. In this way, excessive mirror-gazing will lead to an unhealthy promotion of Self. Consistent with the Narcissus predicament; Self promotes Self, the mind changes the narrative accordingly, and viability for its own sake replaces social intensiveness. In other words, Self creates a commune with itself. This creates a false sense of network that loops. This is inevitable because Self interpretation is how Self defines social viability; it does this by informing the story the mind tells itself. In this way, the mind-informing-mind-narrative is the mirror Self should be gazing into.

Aoife: But unlike Narcissus I am not in love with what I see?

Dad: Self has positive and negative regard for its rendering. Remember, Self promotes items in attention consistent with its *learnt* understanding of social viability; Self can learn to validate its own destruction. Beautiful or ugly, how ever it has learnt to regard it, Self will promote its own image.

Aoife: Mirror, mirror *off* the wall?

Dad: There is a different way to look into a mirror.

Aoife: Which is?

Dad: A baby will laugh at its reflection. It is amused by it, inconsequentially of Self formation. In the absence of Self, the rendering is amazing. Be amazed by what the imagination is capable of in terms of making 'you' substantive. Consistent with my approach also recognise that the rendering is known. This is also astonishing. Astonishment is a default; it is the wonderment awareness manifests consequential to the focusing of it that you are. Revel in astonishment and recognise, obsession and judgement are conditions of Self. You are not Self.

Aoife: A mirror meditation?

Dad: It can be. Look without seeing, and laugh.

Aoife: Is sleep important.

Dad: Yes. Meditation gives-way to consciousness. It is the act of pulling the curtain of Self back to 'reveal' awareness, which is always present. Meditation is awareness seeking awareness and sleep is consciousness becoming only consciousness. Regard deep sleep as the only way to truly experience consciousness knowing *only* itself and knowing you *only* as itself.

Aoife: You mentioned earlier, 'Ego' is a curtain?

Dad: More accurately, ego *powers* Self. Ego keeps the curtain closed that is made of Self. It is a curtain many never peek behind, or they actively 'staple' closed. Consider: *Self is an 'announcement' of social viability and asks that a degree of existential kudos is acknowledged. Just like a curtain in a theatre, it 'anticipates' an authentic character. Is it better to keep the curtain closed and let authenticity be suspected or open the curtain and remove all doubt? Most choose the first option.* Self can be a place where a superficial representation of accolades, pretentions, witticism, relationships, networks, etc. can be 'pinned'. Some of these qualities should be part of the first-impression you hope to make, others are unwanted 'conditions' of Self. But they are all the 'curtain'. For some the idea of pulling the curtain back means 'pulling-aside' who they *think* they are and 'giving-up' their identity. This is reasonable, for many a considerable about of time, struggle and achievement has gone into hanging that Self-curtain and making it look good. However, *it is only a curtain* that exists to 'announce' your social viability.

Aoife: So, ego and Self are not dirty words, but they can get scruffy?

Dad: They become toxic when they are not 'allowed' to fulfill their duties.

Aoife: But they really want to be the captain of the ship?

Dad: They are constantly answering life and death questions; they must have a 'presence'. Consider: *We do not sleep in an ego 'powered' state. We do not have the thought 'item' coming into attention — I am brilliant at sleeping. Deep sleep returns us to our essential nature; there is no purpose for Self.*

Aoife: Are we traveling back in time when we sleep?

Dad: No. *If* consciousness is a plane consisting of infinitesimally small data points, this 'plane' is infinite. Remember: *The finite cannot know the infinite, or more accurately, the infinite knows only itself.* The consciousness 'data-points' become 'available' to us during sleep by means of awareness becoming aware of only itself. Imagine, during our waking moments, consciousness is 'focused' in us like a bird that sits on the ocean. Every instant 'appears' to flow past and is immediate to our attention. Now imagine the bird is soaring high above, the water flow appears slower. If the water is the plane of consciousness, the soaring bird is our deep-sleep 'perspective'. This makes data-points on the plane of consciousness appear to be more available. Consciousness *relaxes* and our perspective shifts making some data appear more accessible. Time is illusionary, if we could 'look' at the past it would appear both static and endless simultaneously: *It is impossible.*

Aoife: What about death?

Dad: Self dies with the body. The defining characteristic of consciousness, or the infinite, is its mindlessness. If you achieve a truly mindless state during meditation the feeling might be that Self has moved aside and your eyes are now a portal through which eternity is *revealed*; regard it as consciousness. It should feel like it occupies a limitless void. Or, if you accept that we are protrusion from the plane of consciousness then you might imagine that during meditation, and sleep, the 'protrusion' you are reduces or becomes less pronounced. Death is the complete collapse of the protrusion. You might think of it as a 'relaxing' of the ripples that *you* once were, on the plane of consciousness. The small entropic role you play changes phase. 'You' now becomes the expanse that is consciousness that knows only itself; an ultimate freedom that is void of memory, time, dimension, sensation, and Self. What then is left of 'you'? Nothing, except flow. We live life understanding that synchronicity leads to a sense of 'flow'. It is an experiencing of consciousness, void of Self. If we accept that entropy is the cooling after an instantaneous disturbance, then flow is correlation. Accept death as a phase change.

Aoife: How do I achieve 'flow'.

Dad: First, 'flow' does not mean your pathway is without obstacle. It means your goal is clear and the challenges are enabling. Imagine a lava *flow*. The centre of the river flows, the periphery of that flow is rock that begins to cool and be 'discarded', increasing disorder and dispersing energy accordingly. When you are in a flow-state you are riding the centre of the flow. However, you will still be 'directed' down a path of least resistance, but the challenges will be consistent with the goal: *For whatever it is you wish to achieve in life be sure the challenges of its attainment are consistent with the nature of its realisation.*

Aoife: So, I must be challenged?

Dad: Yes. The elite sportsperson who 'feels' a sense of flow has *worked* for it. The hundreds of shots taken in training means the three-pointer scored in the game feels second-nature. This is what is meant by - act without action. The more you are not placing the completion of something as an 'item' into attention the less likely it is that Self will promote it. 'Action' describes what Self does when it 'sees' items in attention. 'Act' describes the state of 'looking' that allows for the mind to be blind. In this way, the hours spent practicing have a meditating effect. Or, in other words, Self will learn not to promote the item in attention. The repetition 'teaches' Self that the action exists for its own sake and is of no social-viability importance. This places the athlete into a 'zone'. Or in other words, a mental place void of doubt and other conditions of Self.

Aoife: I sometimes feel that not all flow is flow?

Dad: You may be in an eddy, which only appears to be flow. For example, if you want to be a stand-up comedian, go to open mic rooms and tell jokes in front of strangers, this will lead to flow — eventually. But if you *only* tell jokes online and then expect to become a professional stand-up with no stage-time, don't be surprised if there is no flow. In other words, social media *can* put creative people into eddies, which is only an *appearance* of flow, that potentially stifles growth.

Aoife: Why do some people seem to have things 'fall into place'?

Dad: They know their superpower.

Aoife: Do I have a superpower?

Dad: Yes, but slow down. I do not mean superpower like a motivational speaker, talking at a conference, trying to make you a better salesperson. And I do not mean literal powers of a superhuman kind. Each of us occupies our own space on the spectrum of kinetic energy. We are a protrusion from the *same* plane of consciousness, but we are also an expression of entropy. In other words, if the universe is to continue to change shape (which it must) each of us *must* be a different expression of its source.

Aoife: So, we are the same but different?

Dad: We are one, multidimensional
expression. My 'superpower' concept relates
to an individual's sense of their
giftedness. Firstly, a 'gift' needs only be
a small deviation away from a shared
ability. Secondly, many people are so
familiar with their 'gift' they fail to see
it.

Aoife: How can it be seen?

Dad: Endeavor, with heavy doses of failure.

Aoife: Got it. Why can't some people love?

Dad: Everyone loves. It is fundamental in
the universe. Some people learn to despise
the people they love. So, they develop a
discomfort with the kind of love that is
fundamental. Fundamentally love is meant to
strengthen bonds that encourage
communication which is correlation. Part of
that process is to accept a degree of
dependency. When we are young, we are
dependent on others who may treat us
unkindly. Self will then associate love with
notions of obligation. Then, in adulthood,
once a degree of independence is achieved,
love, without a sense of obligation or
conditions, can be difficult to realise.
Survival requires dependency, we experience
it as love because it is fundamental. When a
child is obliged to love, the adult they
become will engage in love with resentment.
Therefore, some people love-to-hate. They
despise love because they know it to be
obligatory, or in other words, they were
forced to learn to love someone they hate.
When the concept of hate is *loved* that love

is not obligatory because the 'action' of it
is destructive. It creates a revenge
scenario - *I will use love to destroy, in my
mind, the person I was obliged to love when
I was a child.* In adulthood dependency
should become in-dependency and
relationships should be a celebration of
oneness in terms of awareness. However,
adults who love to hate will always be
dependant until they disconnect notions of
obligation from love. They will always be
dependent on *hateful* acts until they
experience unconditional love. Animals
provide love unconditionally; dogs can
retrain a human to love, *love* again.

Aoife: Is life meant to be easy?

Dad: Yes, and active. Destruction in the
universe does not mean destroyed. Your life
should be a constant cycle of reconfiguring
that begins with deconstruction. Therefore,
to make life easy it should be an endeavour.
Life becomes hard when you attempt to
maintain structures and force equilibrium.
It is impossible to make the world
predictable. It is much easier to engage in
a reconfiguring process. Exploring the
transferability of your skills and
experience across industries is an ideal
example. Do not confuse *comfort* with ease.

Aoife: Is there a shortcut?

Dad: There is nothing to cut, go directly.
Remember: *The temporally informed hardware
that is your mind and body cannot know the
infinite, and consciousness can never adopt
a sense of time.* Under the influence of
'shortcuts' the mind can *expand* its

sensitivity and accept a boundlessness inquisitorial state. In this way, the mind becomes more like a blank canvas onto which *interpretations* of consciousness can be projected. But this is not the consciousness that is fundamental; it is more like a Hollywood interpretation. However, some altered state experiences can profoundly enhance developmental reappraisal. When consciousness reconciles with the mind and body mistakes can be made. With 'assistance' the entrenched nature of these 'errors' can be exposed, allowing the origin-self to tell a new story.

Aoife: So, can consciousness *feel*?

Dad: Consciousness does not *feel*, it is not concerned for your pain or torment. Consciousness is the source of the 'mind' and the mind is the source of 'trust' and trust is the most efficient means for continuous processing. Consciousness must learn the limits of the mind and body to initiate this processing. Of course, consciousness does not 'learn' or care or motivate. It may be regarded as the electricity that flows into a computer; it is indifferent and *is* flow. Now imagine this electricity flows the easiest through circuits configured in a cascade. In other words, they are in a state of endless processing like the currents in a stream. Consciousness 'cares' not for the nature of the componentry so long as the cascading continues. In this way consciousness may be imagined as a charged, eternal resource with no intent and seeks only a course of least resistance. If our Self is cascading, as the metaphor suggests, then *flow* will manifest in your life. This does not mean you will win the lottery. First change nothing except the desire to change.

Aoife: Change *change*?

Dad: Remember, Self is constantly seeking 'connectedness' to consciousness. It will attempt to do this by attaining 'things'. For example, a more secure job, a new car, a better relationship. The 'attainment' of these items alleviates the pressure for Self to be goal, or validation orientated. Self is constantly seeking feedback to assess its social viability. The achievement of a socially dynamic objective temporarily 'removes' the *seek* motivation from Self. The absence of external focuses allows for Self to 'sense' its source.

Aoife: It 'allows' Self to dissolve into consciousness?

Dad: Yes, giving us a sense of peace and connectedness. Remember, everything comes from consciousness. The mind, the body, the Self, the child you once were are all 'protrusions' from the plane of consciousness. Consciousness knows only itself and knows you only as itself. Therefore, consciousness is unchanging. This is one means for understanding why the finite cannot know the infinite. Infinite consciousness is not 'tricking' time and has not been given immortal qualities. Consciousness knows *only* itself; it simply has no 'knowledge' of time: *It cannot change*. Without the distraction of external objectives Self 'connects' again with consciousness and is reminded of the sense of freedom it provides. If, however, Self learns that the attainment of validation is a means for generating this 'connectedness', it will come back into 'attention' and you will feel the *seek* drive again. I am asking you to arrest Self at this moment; there is a direct means and it requires *no* change. Or in other words, it requires no validation or ongoing reward.

Aoife: So, I should stop seeking to 'change' my life.

Dad: Yes. Specifically, stop looking at changing the 'items' in your life. Life needs no-*thing.* Remember, everything is illusion-*ary*; illusions do not need a new toaster, or fame, etc. Change your attitude towards the *need* for change. In other words, total freedom is a return of the essential you into a change-*less* state. This is consciousness, unfettered by Self, or the body, or time, or mind, etc. This essential 'you' (informed by time and space and is known as the 'observer') is *not* Self. You might like to imagine consciousness can 'look' through your eyes to see the strange 'time-and-space' dimension your mind and body occupies. When it does this it sees the Self version of you; Self manifests as personality and is illusionary. Reflect: *Imagine your 'eyes' are binoculars. At one end is consciousness looking through, at the other end is 'time-and-space' in which your-Self appears. The binocular body is a 'buffer', or phase-change device, allowing the infinite and the finite to 'connect'. The key point is this, you are not Self, you are not pure consciousness, you are the space between. You are the binocular body 'made' of consciousness. Connectedness is a word that attempts to explain a means by which timelessness can be inferred.*

Aoife: What do you mean by 'direct means'?

Dad: At reconciliation (childhood), as consciousness 'recognises' the limits of mind and body, a *circuit-board* for processing is printed. This is the foundation of Self, I refer to it as the origin-self, it can also be referred to as inner-child. Imagine a computer with a power lead, going into a power-converter that then distributes the power to the components. The 'observer' that we 'essentially' are, is the 'power-converter'. However, imagine it can also add components to the circuit bord towards the creation of an *adult* computer. The power-converter 'uses' this circuit board to manage the 'time-and-space' constraints of the mind and body (which manifests as process dependency). The power-converter, however, is *not* the circuit bord. In other words, you are not Self – a computer is not its circuit bord; without the power-converter, the computer is nothing. To go *directly* means you realise your true nature as the power-converter. Remember: *if consciousness is the electricity flowing into the power-converter then the power-converter and all other parts of the computer are also 'made' of consciousness. Therefore, if you can 'be' the power-converter you have connectedness to the sources of your creation.*

Aoife: So 'connectedness' is like oneness?

Dad: Yes. But remember, it is impossible to
be *one* with everything because everything is
one.

Aoife: Can you explain what you mean by
'reconciliation' again?

Dad: The 'observer' *allows* aspects of Self
to *fuse* together. This is enabled by the
'observer's' third person perspective; much
like a sculptor adding clay to a figure. The
fusing takes place during childhood and is a
response to the story the mind is telling.
The story is constantly being revised by the
mind as Self *learns* to be socially viable.
Remember: *The nature of social viability is
relative; informed by a response to
circumstances.*

Aoife: What about fate?

Dad: It is true that subatomic particles
feel funny about being looked at. Let us
accept, that when observed, particles will
take a 'form' but if no one is looking they
can 'choose' to be formless. Further to
this, particles can behave in a way that
suggests they have knowledge of the future.
'Knowledge' and 'particle', however, are
words that should never be in the same
sentence together. Fate describes the
awareness of the barrier between the
intention of the observed and the effect of
the unobserved. Remember, everything is a
'protrusion' from the plane of
consciousness, including all deterministic
sensitivity. Consciousness is known only to
itself — the entirety of it *is* only itself.
The more we adopt the 'observer' perspective
the more we have a sense that the *normal*

state is, therefore, changeless. Fate is the sensing of timelessness, whereby everything *appears* to manifest at once. In this way, fate is the sensing of correlations *arising* from an unobservable consciousness, and the observable, synchronistic use of the available energy the *arising* creates. It is for this reason that fate feels mysterious; it is not.

Aoife: Do you think there will be a theory of everything?

Dad: Yes. But a theory of everything should, at its core, enable a redefining the theory of everything endlessly. In other words, the destination is a place where processing the processing will lead to a never-ending cycle of processing.

Aoife: Are we all going to the same destination?

Dad: Yes; if entropy, variety, and correlation can be conceived as destinations. It is for this reason that the journey must become the destination. You are then the journey; non-objectified.

Aoife: Why is it harder for some to 'process' their feelings?

Dad: Connectedness to consciousness is the reason. Consciousness 'seeks' processing and processing is inevitable. It is better that you allow for processing consistent with increasing correlations, rather than feeling like external forces are 'bullying' you into change. Where there is a need for processing and no means for its expression flow loops

unstably. In other words, some people have
under-developed Self tools and try to
pervert processing. However, entropy and
variety must increase; a means for
processing will manifest. Then, various
types of stress may emerge and become
default processes. Consciousness cannot
'know' unstable loops; correlations must
expand not 'loop'.

Aoife: Consciousness *prefers* process?

Dad: Remember, consciousness does not *like*
or *feel* anything. Everything is a
manifestation of consciousness and is
therefore consciousness; there is no
separation. In this way, consciousness can
only know itself and knows you as only
itself: *Because you are it-Self; there is
literally no separation between any
consequence of consciousness.* There is,
therefore, no separation between
individuals; we are all the one
consciousness. Remember, consciousness knows
'us' but it knows nothing of 'stuff' and,
therefore, time. The answer to the question
— should there be no-*thing* in the universe,
is yes, and that 'yes' manifests itself as
time. Time is process and, in a way, it is a
process that allows consciousness to
'experience' the universe as static, or an
expression of no-*thing*.

Aoife: But time is not static?

Dad: it is a collection of infinitesimally
short instances. Each instant is
immeasurably short to the extent that any
processing ceases to be present; there are
no *things*. Consider: *The difference between*

*two adjacent instances is, essentially,
meaningless.* Does the water *know* the wave
caused by the stone as something separate
from itself? It would be impossible for it
to investigate any given instant and expect
to see a wave. The universe is the
unknowable wave.

Aoife: Is 'consciousness' in the brain?

Dad: There are aspects of consciousness that
are difficult to explain; it is known as the
'hard' problem. The electrical activity of
the brain can be plotted, the interconnectedness of the components observed and
yet the feeling we have of this activity is
real but apparently unexplainable. In other
words, awareness remains elusive. Imagine
again the computer studying itself: *But this
time it is looking at its own central
processing unit.* After dissections and
replications are made, the *activity* of the
unit may be determined. However, until the
computer accepts that the central processing
unit is 'made-of' consciousness, or as the
metaphor suggests, is made of electricity,
the true nature of the central processing
unit will not be understood.

Aoife: The computer is *made* of electricity
but is unable to conceive the nature of
electricity?

Dad: Yes, this is central to the metaphor.
Any attempt to change, or observe, the
nature of the *electricity* will mean the
computer ceases to exist. Consciousness is
made purely of consciousness: *We are a
protrusion from the plane of consciousness
known to consciousness only as itself.* The

time-*less* is differentiated from the time-*restricted* because of a correlation of infinitesimally small instances. In this way, consciousness is the bedsheet, and we are a bedbug crawling across it; the sheet is infinite. Even though the bedbug cannot 'be' the sheet, I am asking you to imagine that the bedbug is made *of* the sheet. In this way, visualise the timeless nature of consciousness as *still*, and we are ripples across its plane. Every instant is then infinite — it feels like time is flowing: *The instances evolve so rapidly it is beyond our ability to comprehend.*

Aoife: The universe is *unknowable* by consciousness?

Dad: Yes.

Aoife: Why do I feel like my feelings control me?

Dad: 'Feelings' are a condition of the Self that help protect and *advance* Self and its objective towards entropy. In this way feelings are responsive, but they *control* literally nothing. If we accept that *in* consciousness everything exists at once then happiness and sadness, anger and joy, etc are always equally *available*. You could regard it like the fracturing of light. When we see the rainbow, we can focus on the blue or the red. But essentially, they all exist simultaneously and without the fracturing would not be distinguishable. Our ability to fracture emotions gives us the illusion that each feeling is a separate agent. Remember: *Consciousness has no means or need to feel anything.* Emotional responses are a survival mechanism designed to protect the *protrusion* we are from the plane of consciousness. We are illusion-*ary* and fundamentally, so too are our feelings. I am not suggesting you ignore your feelings – they are the canary in the cage, as they arise the story the mind tells itself changes. I am asking you to not be controlled by them by accepting they are a 'condition' of Self.

Aoife: Why then, do we 'fracture' our emotions?

Dad: Our need to process means that we must fracture. Towards processing the imagination will itemise everything including emotions. The fracturing *is* an act of processing. It is an act of de-construction. Which is the most effective means for processing anything; its sectioning manifests its reorganisation. In this way, to be socially viable we must present the world with a story and stories need timelines. Consequently, we are *forced* to separate emotions and put them into a sequence; the timeline allows for one piece of data at one time. Accept that emotions are not 'stopping' and then start again. Their potential to *come-forth* is always present.

Aoife: So social viability is the reason why I feel *controlled* by my feelings?

Dad: Jealousy, anger, sadness, love, etc are conditions of the Self. Self, typically, evolves into a combination of *apparently* toxic, benign and constructive elements. You may regard Self as a carriage driver with a team of horses, a horse called envy, another called love, a horse called anger, etc.

Driving the horses is your origin-self. This
entity is a child, the child you were at a
critical stage of development. Hopefully, in
development this child had moments of
clarity where all the horses were pulling
together, no one horse was doing more than
it needed to, no one horse was encouraged to
lead excessively; for this has consequences.
For example, if the horse called love is
pushed forward and consistently receives no
reward, sycophantic, obsessive, insecurity,
etc traits may characterise your Self later
in life. The rule of entropy dictates that
these problems will attract greater
complexity as Self develops. Recall the
example of obligatory love, it leads to the
loving of the feeling 'hate'. In western
cultures we stop asking who-am-I early in
development forcing our inner-world to seek
stability prematurely; our origin-self then
becomes resistant to change. In this state
your origin-self will seek to manipulate the
'outside' factors to ensure the 'internal'
factors are more predictable, in other
words, to maintain the integrity of the
story the mind tells itself.

Aoife: How does it do that?

Dad: Consider: *The sycophant is drawn
towards the narcissist. One wants to praise
and the other needs it; the integrity of
their narratives are prioritised regardless
of the 'unseen' instability.* Consequently,
people may find themselves in cycles of
abuse. If they hope to *break* the cycle they
must 'revisit' critical moments in their
development; allowing the mind to retell a
different story.

Aoife: How do they do that?

Dad: The inner-child wants love and occupation.

Aoife: Love and joy?

Dad: Self love.

Aoife: Why do people make me angry?

Dad: Other people literally cannot make you angry. *You* are placing anger into your attention.

Aoife: But it feels like they *are* making me angry?

Dad: You are the only one who can place anything into your attention. Or more specifically, only you can choose what is promoted in your attention. Remember, your imagination is placing all the characteristics of your current time and place, and any associated *items* into your attention *constantly*. The unique nature of your Self will determine what is promoted in your attention. Therefore, you choose what is promoted in attention; *Self* chooses to promote anger. Mastery of Self gives you greater power over what 'stays' in your attention.

Aoife: So, nothing 'external' can *make* you angry?

Dad: Anger is important. I use anger when you are placing yourself in harm's way. I will get angry with my Self. Consequently, Self may need to stridently reorder its list

of priorities. Other people, however, cannot
make me angry. In other words, why would I
choose to raise in my attention stress that
I do not own? It is important to note that
when other people want you to feel angry or
sympathetic or frustrated 'for them', they
are asking you to help tell a story that is
not *your* story. Helping someone tell their
story is not *helping,* it is enabling.

Aoife: So, what should I feel for them? Or
what should I 'place into my attention'?

Dad: Relatively? Disappointment, sadness, be
pensive, empathetic, hopeful, etc are
responses that help inform *your* story.
Essentially, reflect on your correlation
with others; this informs your story. Make
your feelings of frustration be specific to
your story and needs. This is, subsequently
the best means for helping others shift
their perspective on their problem; your
story exists as a piece of data to help
redirect their story.

Aoife: Sometimes, it is hard for anger to
not *rise* in attention?

Dad: You can replace the *item* that is anger
with the item that is apple. This is a
direct approach; visualise an apple.

Aoife: Why apple?

Dad: Apple is an idea, an image, a thought,
an object, and a great place to start.
Imagine, I have started a meditation by
asking you to visualise an apple and then I
respond to a text message; you will be
struck by my rudeness. That feeling will

replace the image of the apple; the thought *item* 'inconsiderate' will replace the image *item* 'apple'. Moreover, it appears that *you* placed apple into attention, and *I* replaced it with 'inconsiderate'. The truth is you placed 'inconsiderate' into your attention; it is something I *literally* cannot do. In other words, your imagination placed 'inconsiderate' into your attention and Self *promoted* it over apple. That does not mean you 'imagined' my rudeness; the rudeness is real. The imagination renders everything and places it into attention and Self promotes items consistent with its needs. Obtaining some control over what gets promoted in attention will help reduce the controlling influence of Self.

Aoife: Is it hard to make Self happy?

Dad: Self cannot be happy. If Self was literally a collection of tools in a box, we would accept a box cannot be 'happy'; tools cannot be happy. The effective Self is one that is available but not present; the ineffective Self is one that is present but not available. Or more specifically is not available for you to 'observe'; it exists as a reactor that controls your choices. The essential you, the protrusion you are from the plane of consciousness, should be present. The essential you becomes present when the tools in the Self box each have a place, are organised, are available in equal measure, and the lid shuts tight. The *essential* you can carry the Self box with pride; keen to upgrade a tool or add one as the mistakes you make in life dictate: *Do not be intimidated by the task of updating*

*Self, it is not a sign of weakness - Self is
not who you are.*

Aoife: Who am I then?

Dad: You are the *'observer'* of Self, that is
your essential 'you'. The 'observer' is
serine and timeless, wide eyed and
enthralled by processes, that seeks to
express all manner of energy - best
described as communication, that is who
'you' are. It is deep, it is calm.

Aoife: Is *love* a Self 'device'?

Dad: We must not forget that love is a force
in the universe; it is a Self-tool and is
also a way of describing oneness —
consciousness. In this way, love *fuels*
communication. Therefore, given that
consciousness only knows you as itself love
must first be directed to Self.

Aoife: How do I love my Self?

Dad: The first step towards Self-love is to
accept you are the most interesting person
you know. You are, and always will be, the
most interesting person you know because you
are Self *and* consciousness. It is a lifelong
commitment to learn the tool of Self from
the *'observer'* perspective. For many of us
Self is a very heavy curtain that must be
pulled at in a sustained and determined
manner if we are to see behind it and reveal
consciousness. We must also close the
curtain and be the Self sometimes
necessarily; relatively. Self is not a dirty
word; Self is the tool that has enabled your
manifestation. Your management of Self

presents a forest-for-the-tree's
predicament; you will never be presented
with a more fascinating endeavour than to
isolate Self and hone your mastery of it.
Appreciate that life is constantly
presenting you with obstacles that force you
to correct, refine and economise Self. In
this way be a learner for life and see
mistakes as an emerging 'aha' moment.

Aoife: Why does Self get angry when I don't
want it to?

Dad: Self has learnt its obligations. Accept
it is circumstantially affected. Accept that
you are a traveller. Anger, manipulation,
denial, etc may be indicators of process
deficiencies; Self is a data processor.
However, there is a perception issue:
*Feeling that some 'thing', an external
factor, has made you angry is inaccurate.*
Others who 'see' you being angry, perceive
it as your current *internal* state.
Suggesting that anger can exist externally
and internally simultaneously; this is not
possible. Anger must build connections
between people. Much like fear, anger is a
response to a threat that may require an
immense amount of data to be processed very
quickly. It is best understood as a warning
process - a flare gun in the Self toolbox.
You may feel that you have no control over
anger. Often anger can be corralled by
asking in the moment 'to what extent is
there a threat to life?'

Aoife: And if that does not work?

Dad: The *only* purpose of anger is to stop
your toddler from grabbing at saucepans

sitting on the stove top, or to stop them from walking too close to the cliff's edge, etc. Anger is learnt early; recall the toddler you once were throwing a tantrum in the shopping centre. Of course, the toddler is expected to learn that frustration need not escalate into anger. However, frustration will always become anger if the child never 'observes' other processing options. So then, what to do when anger is too 'readily' available? Trying to explain to your angry Self some notion of process deficiency is like forcing a computer to stop the flow of its own electricity. Instead recognise that the anger is a 'process' and invite it into your attention completely. Then recognise that it *must* lead to other processing. Remember: *Anger, love, regret, joy, etc, exist simultaneously.* Go directly to another place on the emotion spectrum. Anger is a protection tool; let anger become nurture. Nurture is a teaching tool; let nurture create consequences.

Aoife: To go *directly*? Harder than it looks?

Dad: In the heat-of-the-moment it is not easy. Communication is necessary; anger must *practice* talking to nurture. In this way communication is a process first and is then a means for understanding. Engaging in any kind of processing will have an immediate reconciling influence: *The more an individual experiences life as a journey of discovery the more synchronised they become with the fundamental nature of the universe.* In other words, nothing ends. All emotions are *always* present. Practice breaking down the channel walls that make it appear as if emotions are separate 'things' with end points. If it helps, imagine anger taps nurture on the shoulder and says 'any suggestions?' Or, imagine you remove the battery from the anger tool and put it into the nurture tool. Also accept, that anger isolated does not achieve anything; it is designed to respond to situations that present real, physical danger. If your child is playing with fire get angry, if they spill paint in the carpet get consequential.

Aoife: I liked the tool analogy. Can I put the same battery in different Self tools?

Dad: Yes, it is called ego. Ego means 'I', but it also describes a strengthening quality, a power that reinforces who we *think* we are, or that promotes Self. There is 'you' and there is a Self which you know as personality. Seeing Self as a set of tools allows you to step back from Self and see it for what it is. Visualising ego as the battery pack that powers the Self tools allows you to understand ego as essential: *The tools of Self exist exclusively to enable your interaction with other people.*

Aoife: So, I use Self to talk to other Selfs?

Dad: Yes. More accurately, you have created a Self that interacts with other created Selfs. Self is learnt, this is central to understanding ego.

Aoife: I do not remember learning Self?

Dad: That is correct, you cannot remember when you started using the anger tool, the patience tool, the sympathy tool, or when

you started filling up your Self toolbox.
Self is learnt in an *acquired* manner;
indirectly.

Aoife: When did I *acquire* ego?

Dad: Ego is the battery pack powering all
your Self tools; it has always been there.
The only motivation of Self is to source
what is necessary to ensure your social
viability. You first experience ego as
exclusively a 'me' only motivator; it exists
to facilitate your immediate needs excluding
all other considerations. It then develops
'we' intentions. Self begins to realise that
a support network is necessary for survival;
this includes immediate family and
significant others. The subsequent
interactions are essential social viability
training. This is most commonly known as
attachment; psychopaths fail to develop this
sense of the village. Incidentally:
*Psychopaths learn to simulate behaviours
consistent with an abiding sense of 'other';
they are unsophisticated puppet masters of
Self*. Ultimately, however, ego must develop
an 'us' dimension. The well-adjusted ego has
a well-placed sense of community beyond the
village. It is characterised by empathy, a
big-picture awareness and, most importantly,
a finish-what-it-starts determination.
Collectively, Self tools become personality,
which you use to interact with others; you
use it for social activity exclusively.
Personality is the way you promote your
collection of Self tools; that *promotion* is
powered by ego.

Aoife: So, personality is an ego performance
directed by me?

Dad: Personality is certainly created by you *circumstantially.* If you know how to manipulate the tools that make up personality effectively it *can* acquire 'targeting' qualities. In other words, it becomes superficial, but this is unsustainable. personality is unsustainable as a performance used to manipulate others. This is how Psychopaths look at personality; it does not end well. Personality is 'directed' by the *'observer'* you essentially are, but the 'observer' only observes, it cannot *literally* direct. The mind, enabled by the imagination, receives data from the 'observer' point-of-view and can change the story it writes for itself, that *stars* your personality.

Aoife: The mind is not *directed* by the 'observer', but it benefits from the bigger-picture point-of-view it provides?

Dad: Yes. This is what is meant by 'getting perspective'. This is a common way people describe problem-solving; it is often associated with taking time-out from a task or putting a problem aside indefinitely. Most people do not have an active sense of the 'observer' and therefore make instinctual decisions to put a problem aside; this can lead to procrastination. The direct approach I am describing allows you to 'step' into the 'observer' *position* in the moment. Or more accurately to *always* be the 'observer' and see Self as a puppet directed by the mind.

Aoife: Adopting the 'observer' *position* is like hitting a reset button.

Dad: More like being the Producer of a film, not the Director.

Aoife: How do I create an authentic personality?

Dad: You must understand the true purpose of ego: *Self and the personality it becomes, must build community; this constructive work is powered by ego.* 'Build community' means, build a network that sustains *you*. This confuses the true purpose of ego: *Ego is a, help-yourself-by-helping-others proposition, not a help-Self-help-itself tool.*

Aoife: So, I must build?

Dad: Yes. Display your tools in the showcase that is your personality. Plug in the ego, then say to yourself, I will build. I will not lure; I will not trick or deceive; I will build. This aligns the function of your Self tools with the fundamental nature of the universe; this is the definition of authenticity.

Aoife: So, 'process' and be happy?

Dad: Yes and learn to love complexity. Complexity will emerge and is central to an ontological focus on processing. The 'processing' is entropy and must increase. Processing creates correlations which will become a map filled with interconnectedness. By combining two simple *agents* the entire complexity of the universe will emerge. The simple or direct *way* includes the appreciation of complexity not the harbouring of it. Neglected processing and its impact on community is burdensome and is an attempt to limit entropy; it is impossible. Mental health care workers exist for a reason and understand the need for *processing*.

Aoife: Are algorithms controlling us?

Dad: Algorithms are not new. Our mind is an algorithm generating machine: *It creates a program made of Self components that are expressed in a character form that we know as personality.* Attention will have 'data' — sadness, new car, ambition, pair of shoes, love, etc placed into it by the imagination. Mind is 'created' as Self begins to promote bits of this data. For most people, the *promotion* includes the placement of Self into a dominate position. In other words, attention is a tool used to focus on data coming from the imagination that is then promoted to the mind by Self. 'Mind' is a way of describing the data's arrangement into an algorithm, that for most people, allows Self to become possessive of the narrative subsequently created.

Aoife: 'Mind' is *just* a word?

Dad: It does not describe anything literal. But it is precisely understood relative to the purposes of Self. The word 'mind' can be used to describe a system that writes the story for the Self that it is also creating; that becomes, hopefully, an effective personality show.

Aoife: *hopefully?*

Dad: Personality is the character created by the mind to express or display to the world the essential ingredients of Self; *hopefully* worthy of replicating with the sharing of genes. Unfortunately, Self is acquired, or 'created' indirectly and mostly circumstantially. The mind is telling itself a story using the data available and relies on Self to *vet* the data first. It is the task of the imagination to provide 'real-time' feedback on the social effectiveness of Self. Self may then adjust what it promotes in attention; the *mind* will make changes to the *algorithm* accordingly.

Aoife: So, the algorithm is updated continuously?

Dad: Yes. Your mind is the first social media tool you should seek to understand. Imagine your mind is an app, feeding you a version of your-Self that fits into a story. The story is written by the mind with data promoted by Self in attention. The story is your 'feed'. Social media platforms want you to stay 'logged in'. Likewise, your mind wants to secure its dependence on Self: *It is easy for Self to be over-promoted, especially when threats to our survival are exaggerated.* Due to a myriad of issues, most people are in a Self-dominance state; they believe Self is 'who' they are. This is not the fault of the mind; the mind is a committed processor brought into existence by Self.

Aoife: What is the cause of an over-promoted Self?

Dad: Often, circumstances. Imagine, at some critical stage, your origin-self was required to over-use compliance, attention seeking, pleading, etc to acquire information towards creating a compliment of Self tools. This desperation, like an addiction, created a skewed definition of social viability; Self then provides the mind with limited choices.

Aoife: What can be done?

Dad: Hopefully, information received from the imagination (as it renders data emerging in the mind's story) will have a 'corrective' influence but that is conditional on the nature of the Self: *Fear of processing failure causes Self to 'override' or obscure any sense of consciousness.* The village is diversity, in development a person must hear many voices.

Aoife: I wish I could log off from my *mind?*

Dad: Understanding your mind as an algorithm generator means you can treat it like the app it essentially is. Let your imagination render the idea of 'logging off' that then can be promoted by Self; the mind will then write its *dissolution* into the story. What are you when you are not your thoughts?

Aoife: Was that question rhetorical? What should I be looking for?

Dad: Nothing, for there is nothing to 'see'. The world is illusionary. Recall the barnacles on the driftwood analogy. The *essential* you is the timeless force that is the driftwood, Self is the barnacles and

plants that grow on it; combined they
'express' a personality. Now remove the
driftwood, the 'personality' disperses. Now
imagine that the barnacles were a literal
extension of the wood; each element
connected to the core by a thread of
consciousness. This thread is massless and
timeless and knows the elements as itself.
If the driftwood *core* is then removed the
'personality' not only disperses it
literally ceases to exist. The extension of
this metaphor asks you to accept that the
wood, the barnacles and the 'connective'
elements are all *made* of the 'wood'.

Aoife: So, to look at who *I* really am means
'I' would cease to exist?

Dad: Central to the idea of an illusionary
world is the perception we have of matter.
Imagine an atom with electrons etc. whizzing
around the nucleus. The orbit of the
particles defines the boundary of the atom,
there is no atom 'wall' as such, and for the
most part an atom *appears* to be mostly
'empty'; it is not, 'empty' is impossible.
The strict movement of particles around a
nucleus is the reason why something feels
solid. Essentially, the 'patterns' of energy
that define the atoms that make up your
finger is incompatible with the particle
orbit patterns in the atoms of a keyboard,
for example. It is the incompatibility that
creates a 'sense' that something is solid.
In other words, the vibratory nature of the
orbiting particles creates the *illusion* that
things are substantive or 'real'. The
apparent solidity of the material world will
'trick' you into believing there is nothing
beyond the physical world. We must activate

other ways of knowing. First, accept that 'seeing' is a rendering process and 'looking' is a *knowing* process. The 'I' you truly are is *known,* it is not *rendered.* Consider: *If there is nothing to know beyond the material world quantum physicists can put the Hadron Collider back in it's box and go home.*

Aoife: What about meditation?

Dad: Do it as a means of *falling* into a mind-blind state, almost as if by accident. The two key aspects of the meditation are 1. the dissolving of Self and its *item* focus, and 2. to disconnect from the mind and its union with Self. A word of warning: *Meditation can be an intensive dissociative experience; Self is realised as separate. It allows you to 'observe' Self as a 'composition' exposing the nature of its authenticity; your sensitivity towards inauthenticity becomes heightened. However, Self cannot remain detached; meditation may disconnect Self but it must also help to reconnect it again. The reconnected Self is one over which you have renewed control and allows you to be authenticity sensitive. In other words, you risk having your enjoyment of reality TV shows and B-grade rom-coms destroyed. Bad acting is, essentially, the rendering of an unsophisticated personality. Also, you may become alienated. Your friends may struggle with your newfound inability to tolerate unsophisticated renderings of Self. However, of greater consequence will be the growing awareness you have for the propensity of people to be governed by Self.* Before any kind of awakening comes an understanding of Self, and its powerful

ability to pervade attention and obscure
awareness.

Aoife: So, I must try *not* to be Self?

Dad: Forcing anything is the opposite of
meditation. The way *is* 'direct', but the
approach needs clearing; this is achieved
indirectly. Remember, we must fall into
awareness, almost as if by accident. In this
way, trying to 'not' be or do something is
contradictory. For instance, I will not ask
you to 'remove' items from your attention as
other approaches suggest. They ask you to
create a blank-mind-state, which is nothing
more than a redefining of a focus on *items*.
Blankness is an 'item'. Ultimately, we must
dissolve any focusing on items. Accept that
everything comes from consciousness
including our ability to objectify
awareness.

Aoife: Is this meditation difficult?

Dad: No; do not be intimidated. I am laying
the foundations for an extremely accessible
meditative experience. This meditation
attempts to reveal something that has always
been with you; and then asks you to *live* for
it. I suggest you make meditation a regular
part of your life. It is good to practice
maintaining a perspective on Self; which is
a key dimension of my approach.

Aoife: Is this where the meditation begins?

Dad: Yes. However, meditation is the
destination. Do not regard this meditation
as having a beginning. Remember: *A focus on
items such as floors, walls, chairs,*

clothing, sadness, sensations, destinations, etc is a 'condition' of an item focused Self; we must free ourselves from a focus on items. In this way we must accept consciousness knows only itself and knows you only as itself. Make yourself comfortable, your eyes can be open or closed. I conduct this meditation with my eyes open; the closed eye state expands my attention allowing for external and internal data sets to be promoted. This makes *more* items available to the mind; my approach is mind-*less*. Instead, open your eyes and attempt to 'look' without *seeing*. Initially, however, closing your eyes may be helpful. The first step is to direct attention on to itself.

Aoife: I place attention into attention?

Dad: Yes. Ultimately attention can be used to look upon itself, or more specifically, look at its origin.

Aoife: How?

Dad: By using the imagination. The imagination is constantly echo-defining our environment to provide data to the mind so it can continue to create the story it tells itself. In this way the imagination can be *used* to redirect the story, or attention inwards so it can dissolve. We begin with the body - imagine you are in a point-of-view position. To do this, first sit comfortably, eyes open. Then stand up, try to be aware of the experience - the physical motions involved, changes to your centre of gravity, other sensation, etc; then sit again. Now, *imagine* standing and introduce as much detail as possible: *Imagine the act of standing in as much kinaesthetic detail as possible.* Closing your eyes may be helpful; the focus should be on what the body feels when it stands and not on what the eyes see.

Aoife: Why exclude what I see?

Dad: Visualisation is the imagination *objectifying* the world. The first step towards removing a focus on items is to focus on what else exists when objects are not in focus. When you search for a light switch in the dark, your fingers are 'given' greater sensitivity. In this way, a focusing on other sensory experiences begins the separation process.

Aoife: What is being separated?

Dad: Self — from its dominate position. We are, essentially, blindfolding Self or, dimming the light of attention. Remember: *Mind-blind is a way of describing the turning-off of the image creator that Self relies on to do its job.* Awareness of the body is essential; it is the tea-leaves in the cup. Our body captures data that reveals to what extent we are trapped by Self.

Aoife: Is this a muscle relaxation exercise?

Dad: No. That is a different approach. I am asking you to 'work' with your imagination first, so it may dissolve. Now, imagine again the act of sitting, recall it with as much detail as possible. Now close your eyes and imagine you are sitting at a café by the beach and there is a cool breeze. As you sit

there in the cool breeze you remember this
moment when you were here with me or reading
this 'talk'; picture it in as much detail as
possible. Now open your eyes and notice any
change to your perceived experience; you
might have a different sense of being
present.

Aoife: Am I now in an imagined world?

Dad: The 'world' *is* illusionary. More
accurately, however, you are mastering your
imagination and revealing it to be a tool
that 'renders' *reality*. It is not just
something used for you to draw a picture of
a Unicorn or create worse-case-scenarios in
your head. It 'maps' the world for us in
close detail instant by instant: *It is
mostly occupied with the 'creation' of
apparently mundane aspects of your perceived
existence. The imagination is a canvas upon
which we paint the picture that is the story
our mind tells itself.* In other words, Self
uses information from the imagination to
'dress' you for the part it wants you to
play in society; this meditation attempts to
remove the costume.

Aoife: I do feel slightly more 'present'.

Dad: Good. It is important to note that
these meditations are walking you towards
revealing something that has always been
'there'. There is nothing *new* to 'show' you.
In this way, be aware of the subtleties in
feeling as Self begins to dissolve. The
sense of consciousness we are in search of
is something that *is* close to the surface;
an awakening might happen unwittingly. Be
wary of those who lead you on a path to

awareness promising a mind altering, explosively aware experience. The path is direct because there is no path: *We must see Self for what it is so it may dissolve to reveal a 'pure' contentment that is no distance from us; it feels timeless and formless.*

Aoife: Now I am more present, what next?

Dad: Focus on 'present'. What is 'presence'?

Aoife: I am not sure. Should I feel there is less happening in my mind?

Dad: More accurately, imagine mind has been put in the backseat. Feel it closely. *Presence* is about 'time'. I am not suggesting it takes *time* to be 'present'. Remember, the way is direct. Being present means to *forget* time. Our beachside café meditation attempts to trick the imagination into directing our attention to a place without time.

Aoife: It is difficult to conceive?

Dad: Then take a moment to imagine your origin-self; it is timeless. Timelessness *is* the child within. In your memory 'lives' the child you were once; they do not respond to time.

Aoife: Then what?

Dad: The child is 'play' dependant. It becomes *immersed* in tasks; time is disregarded. Essentially, the origin-self is pure 'presence'. It can help you reconnect to a pure sense of focus.

Aoife: The image I have of my Self as a child is unstable?

Dad: Remember, this is an act of your imagination. Go back to the café, create the 'story' again. Open your eyes and feel a greater sense of presence.

Aoife: The child is then more easily rendered?

Dad: Hopefully. Close your eyes and see the child you *are*.

Aoife: The child is not 'playing'?

Dad: The child might come to you unhappy, or dejected, or disenchanted, etc. Consider: *This meditation is not therapy; there is a way to address the needs of the child which interest me. But psychologists and other mental health professionals exist for a reason; find the right one for you.* Picture your Self *as* the child; place them in the centre of a room. Then let the child draw, read, play with dolls, Lego, cars, paints, etc. *As* the child let yourself be consumed by the task. Remember: *This is an act of the imagination; indirectly you are informing the story the mind is writing for itself. Slowly we are isolating Self; we start by 'seeing' its origin.*

Aoife: Does this relate to consciousness?

Dad: Yes, Self obscures awareness; isolating it allows for it to be sidelined. The *child* is timeless, and this associates directly with consciousness.

Aoife: So, meditation is time travel?

Dad: This type of meditation is an act of
the imagination that helps *remove*
obstructions. Remember: *Consciousness knows
only itself and knows you only as itself. It
also knows time only as itself. Or more
accurately because it knows only itself it
cannot know time.* Our experience of time is
a consequence of infinitesimally short
instances racing past. The more one moment
is like the next the more we experience a
sense of timelessness.

Aoife: Meditation makes one moment
indistinguishable from the next?

Dad: All moments are indistinguishable from
the next. Remember: *The difference between
two adjacent instances is, essentially,
meaningless.*

Aoife: And so, the child is a
personification of infinity?

Dad: Yes, an objectifying of it. Which helps
us connect to notions of timelessness and
subsequently awareness. The child who is
'absorbed' in a task, is completely consumed
by it, beyond the ability to respond to
time. The child who is fully engaged in a
task do not fear the judgement of their
Unicorn picture, are not distracted by the
traffic or questions about enlightenment.
They are not fettered by momentary
distractions — they are purely 'processing'
the task: *They know themselves only as a
'processor' and know the processing only as
themselves.*

Aoife: When the child is 'focused' I feel a release of tension through my core, but it also feels energising?

Dad: Good. Remember, we are 'using' the imagination to dissolve the imagination and, subsequently, Self. With practice, we can go directly to this tension-free feeling and sustain it effortlessly. You are on the path.

Aoife: But then sometimes it is hard to engage the 'child'?

Dad: Be mindful of the child's needs and seek professional help accordingly. Remember, I am giving you a way of seeing Self. I am asking you to accept that Self is not who *you* are. If you accept this approach, I can help you see the purpose of Self and what makes it up; including the nature of its origin. The child needs nurturing, or in other words, *you* need nurturing. Reimagining the *child* means you can rewrite the mind-creating-mind story. Let the child be the enthralled 'processor' they once were or have always wanted to be. Like any child they want to play and be happy; a step in any direction away from that and the child is lost. It is true for many that their inner-child is disengaged; it teaches Self to promote bitterness, regret, jealousy, etc.

Aoife: Can you explain the muscle relaxation meditation method?

Dad: The body 'captures' data that reveals how *trapped* a person might be by Self. This

will manifest in tension and dis-ease. This
meditation helps see Self for what it really
is by understanding what it is doing to the
body. Lie on the floor and close your eyes.
Let your attention bring your feet into
awareness. Focus on any tension in your feet
and let the muscles release. Now your
calves, release any tightness or muscle
activity. Now your thighs, etc.

Aoife: Why wasn't I aware of the tension
before?

Dad: It is difficult to describe the truly
pervasive nature of Self. Self *is* the
survival instinct. It is priming you for a
response to your situation, or more
specifically, society. The body must be
ready to either stand and defend, run and
hide or mediate.

Aoife: How can the *body* mediate?

Dad: The mind is the body. All thoughts and
actions are items brought into attention by
the imagination, mostly for the purposes of
Self. All communication is a subtle
combination of gestures, words and habitude.
Self makes these into items with apparently
distinguishable qualities; combined they
form a personality. In this way, mediation
can be more about 'how' the communication is
conducted.

Aoife: Is the muscle relaxation meditation
an inside-outside approach?

Dad: It might feel like that. However, there
is no separation. This realisation is what
makes this version of a muscle relaxation

meditation different. It is important that you no longer conceive thoughts and sensations as existing in the mind. Remember, the 'mind' only comes into existence to assemble, in any given instant, narrative elements. Mind arranges these elements consistent with the story it tells itself.

Aoife: My body can 'think'?

Dad: It is all one. Once you have focused on every muscle group in the body, reassess your entire body and release any residual tension. The best way to do this is to imagine a vivid white light passing through your body from head to toe, as the light moves through it 'deactivates' your muscles. Now *think* of a child reaching up to a hot saucepan and note the tension shift in your body; it may only be very subtle. You will note that the body 'primes' *instinctively* in response to the thought; it is beyond your 'conscious' control. In this way the body is merely an extension of the brain. In other words, the mind and body are one.

Aoife: The image of the burnt child has ruined the meditation?

Dad: Then rewrite the story. Imagine you step forward and stop the child; now let your body relax again. Outside of awareness the mind is writing a new story for itself constantly. So, do what the mind does, use the imagination to rewrite a new story. If it helps, imagine the vivid white light again traveling head to toe, switching-off muscles as it passes through them.

Aoife: And what about the inner-child?

Dad: Good question. Remember the version of
the inner-child who is fully engaged? Recall
the tension released at that time of
engagement; that was the feeling of Self-
dissolving away from the mind and body.

Aoife: Why?

Dad: The mind-body is created in childhood,
and it is a union that occurs before Self is
developed. In this early stage a rudimentary
Self emerges, defined by one characteristic,
it is *endeavouring*. By using the imagination
and re-'engaging' the inner-child Self-
returns to this one-dimensional state. In
other words, the Self that the adult version
of you knows, that is constantly using
attention to obscure awareness, has been
dissolved.

Aoife: And how does this connect to the
muscle relaxation meditation.

Dad: Relax your muscles, let the light
travel through your body. Now imagine the
inner-child again, see them with the doll, a
book, pens and paper, etc. Now snatch the
object of their endeavour away from them.
Feel the response acutely, note the change
in your muscles. You *will* feel a tingle in
your fingers as the adrenaline is released.
You may experience a feeling of sadness or
anger. Note the physical response; tears
well, fist forms, jaw tightens, etc. Then
relax again.

Aoife: Can I imagine the light again.

Dad: Not so fast. Consider for a moment, what if your inner-child is like a foundation version of your Self and is always present? Like an upside-down pyramid, the inner-child is the *projection* point for the pyramid that all augmentations and additions feed from and are forever connected to?

Aoife: The 'child' changes, everything changes?

Dad: Yes, potentially. The muscle relaxation meditation demonstrates that mind and body are one. Managing tension in the body *is* managing tension in the mind. The relaxation approach also enhances the comprehension of the origin-self or inner-child. This then allows for Self to recede. Self can then be 'seen' as the survival tool it is; the mind and body should not be something Self *possesses* towards its own survival. Also, the muscle relaxation exercise can be used to release the grasp Self has on our instincts.

Aoife: What are instincts?

Dad: Lessons taught by the *now*.

Aoife: Should I trust my instincts?

Dad: Only if you understand the difference between intuition and superstition.

Aoife: Which is?

Dad: Intuition is taking your lessons from now, superstition is fear. Superstition is letting the past teach you how to be controlled.

Aoife: Controlled by what?

Dad: Self. Self will promote items in attention that illicit endocrinal responses creating the illusion of intuition. For many people instinctual experiences are actually fear responses. Self will counterfeit instinctual or intuitional responses.

Aoife: How do I know when Self is 'hacking' my instincts?

Dad: Instinct and intuition do not associate with the past. They describe the process of receiving instruction from the 'now'.

Aoife: How do I take lessons from the *now*?

Dad: Most people take their lessons from the past. This is an extremely common mistake. First, we must accept that the past does not exist. Even in the light of the work done by the imagination, in waking and dream states, to render *everything,* we must realise the impermanence of the past. In this way, memories are not lessons, they are bits of data for the mind to use in the story it tells.

Aoife: We learn nothing from the past?

Dad: The lessons learnt from the past are known as, traditions. Traditions, however, are not intuitional. Tradition is a guide that points to where the path is; and the path is the destination. The *now* teaches us how to stay on it. To put tradition in the

driver's seat is living in response to fear.
This may not be an understanding easily
accepted by most. In this way it is
important to acknowledge fear is a means by
which Self maintains control. Intuition is,
therefore, understood as the act of
interpreting information from the present;
it is not mystical. It is *presence*. We are
often forced into being *present* when a
moment is informed by stress. Essentially,
being *present* describes the promotion of
data contained in the *now*. This is because
the data of the past and the future cannot
associate. Reflect: *We cannot program a*
fruit picking machine to locate fruit based
on the past arrangement of the fruit; every
season the fruit will present differently on
the tree.

Aoife: What is *now* 'data'?

Dad: To learn the lesson of now we must look
at now exclusively. We understand now to be
everything contained within an instant.
Instantaneously, information is made
available. This information consists of
correlations, the tangential nature of
which, allows for everything in the universe
to manifest including entropy. Instant by
instant awareness *knows* the protrusions that
we are arising from it is indiscernible from
itself. Instinct can then be understood, as
a sensitivity of the entropic nature of any
given instant. In other words, if any
quivering in the vibration that is the
fundamental expression of entropy is
detected, it must be corrected. When we feel
this extremely subtle entropic imbalance,
the *now* is 'suggesting' a refocusing on the
available data. The 'gut' feelings we have

are simply a invitation issued by our true
nature to be present. Consider: *Our
instincts are most active in conditional
situations. Conditions attempt to reduce
variables; an unsophisticated expression of
energy is unsustainable.*

Aoife: Can you explain how the mind creates
a story for *itself* again?

Dad: The imagination 'places' *items* into
attention as it echo-defines your place in
time and space.

Aoife: What are 'items'?

Dad: Any thought, word, image, emotion,
sensation, etc. The imagination 'places'
items into attention so the mind can create
the 'story'. In other words, this 'data'
informs the decisions you make. For most
people these decisions are consistent with
the needs of Self. Therefore, if allowed to,
Self will 'promote' *items* for the purposes
of its own survival.

Aoife: How does it do that?

Dad: It is constantly 'scanning' the data
the imagination places into attention. If
Self is well adjusted, it will 'promote'
data that helps ensure social viability. If
it is not well adjusted, it will have a
poorly conceived sense of social viability.

Aoife: Is the body and item?

Dad: Yes, it is the first of all items. Self
must be understood as an item defining tool.
It is true that the imagination renders all

items, but it is the process of promotion that means they become distinctive. This is work Self does consistent with its *training*. For example, the item 'anger', and its subsequent sensual manifestations can be objectified. Any sensation, therefore, lends itself to objectification. The divisible nature of most objects makes their management conceivable, but it also makes the identification of other significant objects more difficult. Singularly, the body. Our physical carriage is burdened with the task of enabling processing, consistent with the activity of the universe, and is the first of all items we bring into attention. We witness this most obviously when a newborn child begins the process of understanding its own physical apparatus. In many ways a baby appears to be confused by the nature of its physical ability and appearance. It is possible, at a stretch, to imagine the baby is possessed by an entity that appears to have no understanding of physical constraint; such is the nature of the infant's clumsiness. The body comes into attention subtly and early in life; we quickly forget its objective qualities. Accept that the body is an item and behaves in attention like any other item. Be aware of how it is promoted by Self. For example, believing you are having a bad-hair-day is a consequence of Self promoting the item known as *body*. The first item rendered by the imagination is the body, consequently it is the item it most proficiently objectifies. In this way, a new understanding of physical awareness needs to be encouraged; you are the 'observer' of items, not their possession.

Aoife: So, the imagination places 'items', including the *body,* into attention?

Dad: Then the mind creates a decision-cascade. Each decision is like a plot-point on a story timeline. The story *must* be 'created'; it is not a cataloguing of reactions. The mind will create a story consistent with the needs of Self and the personality it manifests. Remember: *The imagination echo-defines the story as it is being told; this data is made available to Self. Self may make small changes to its promotion activity; the mind then tells a slightly different story. Because of this feedback we describe the story as something the mind is telling 'itself'.* 'Mind' is a way of describing how data is arranged, it is not a literal thing.

Aoife: Does this relate to meditation?

Dad: Yes. First, 'attention' is a *fixed* focusing. In other words, imagine it is a light that is stationary, and the imagination *brings* data to it. Self filters this data for its own purposes first before the mind creates the story. Therefore, Self can very easily distort or exaggerate this 'data'. In meditation we try to stop Self being so dominant or *possessive* of the data. We try to realise that the only *things* that can ever really be placed before attention is whatever is immediately in your time and space; this is the essence of living-in-the-moment. Those *things* need to be seen for what they fundamentally are first, before an ill-formed Self distorts them; this can be achieved through meditation.

Aoife: And secondly?

Dad: Any 'image' that exist in your attention is an *item* and *everything* is an item. The imagination *visualises* because it must give an item an 'apparent' form first before it can echo-define it.

Aoife: What about *dreamt* items?

Dad: Or items that appear when under the influence of substances?

Aoife: Indeed?

Dad: In your waking state the bandwidth of attention is narrow, and the items placed into it come from an *external* sources. In your dream state the bandwidth of attention is wider allowing you to merge many item *types* together. These items exist in your memory or, in other words, exist *internally*. They are a mashing together of internal and external *renderings*; consistent with the story the mind has been telling itself. Under the influence of 'substances', or in an *altered* state, the bandwidth is wider again allowing all internal and external data to exist at once; in a way *not* necessarily consistent with the mind-telling-mind story. The waking, dream and altered states are *item* focused; my approach to meditation asks you to *dissolve* items. In other words, for example, hallucinogenic drugs *reveal* to Self a new set of objectifiable data; this is the opposite of meditation and blocks the way to awareness: *Do not be mind-more, be mind-less.* In an altered state you may see the face of God, or touch his beard, but be aware that the imagination is rendering 'notions' of God. You may also 'see' a *mystical* connection between people and things, but you are objectifying *preconceived* connections. When you 'see' or 'sense' *any* item, it means attention has received it from the imagination.

Aoife: So, be aware of objectifying anything, it is the opposite of 'awareness'?

Dad: You can look at it that way. However, do not try to 'remove' items; that is an objective act. Being Self-aware is the first step towards understanding Self for its item focus.

Aoife: The more I learn about Self the more I do not care for it?

Dad: Once we have some control over what is promoted in attention, we can begin to comprehend the controlling influence of Self; but it must be loved. Eventually we must look at what Self makes vivid in attention without fear and learn to love Self for its intentions. Remember: *Consciousness knows Self only as itself; 'everything' emerges or is a protrusion from consciousness.*

Aoife: Sometimes Self is hard to love 'for its intentions'?

Dad: Allow fear, or loss, or inadequacy, etc to sit in attention and be pure in its nature, not 'contaminated' with other itemised tangents of thought. This is the first step towards being *grateful* to Self. Eventually, Self may need to relearn what to 'promote'; but start by *fully* receiving what it currently makes vivid.

Aoife: But I will be rewarding Self with my acknowledgement?

Dad: We do not want to *reward* Self for over-promoting anger, for example. But we want to *know* the true nature of the anger so we can *determine* the true reason why Self must promote it. Understanding the *specific* source of the anger creates perspective. Acceptance then exists as an item to be promoted by Self. Anger is displaced and *moves-down* the hierarchy of promotable items.

Aoife: So, Self is not the enemy?

Dad: Self is your *child*. Consider: *Self promotes items in your attention like a cat that brings you gifts of half-eaten mice and birds. The cat is being purposeful and wants its survival-abilities to be recognised. Likewise, when Self 'highlights' negative items in attention Self is being purposeful, towards your survival. The purpose is ill-informed, but Self only knows what it has learnt; it knows itself as only what it has learnt.* Begin to love what it puts into attention and Self will begin to promote items less desperately: *At the core of all things that Self makes vivid in attention is a powerful sense of social viability; the central aspect of which is the need to survive.* The circumstances of your life may have given Self motivations it erroneously intends are central to survival. Learn to love these intentions. Or in terms of the metaphor, when the cat displays its kill

give it some affection, and then begin
giving it unsolicited attention and it will
less likely make *gruesome* displays to garner
affection. Likewise, Self might make doubt,
for example, vivid in attention. Thank Self
for its efforts, look at the doubt closely
and see it as Self simply doing its job
well. Then continue more and more to invite
Self to drag-its-kill into your attention;
this is the essence of loving *your*-Self. It
is all ultimately an act of love because it
all protrudes from consciousness from which
the concept of unity itself arises.

Aoife: Will my relationship with Self always
be difficult?

Dad: It is true that Self holds a strong
position. It appears to constantly want to
inform the story the mind tells; it often
does this by over-promoting or exaggerating
the data. I am trying to give you tools to
be the 'observer' of Self and begin to
comprehend why it promotes items in
attention. However, Self can be dominant for
decades; its position is not easily
redefined. Therefore, it is important to
understand that Self will seek to maintain
control and that's why it must be loved and
not despised.

Aoife: Are there any other consequences?

Dad: If it is not valued Self can *attach* to
a part of your body. Some tension-release
style meditations are an acknowledgement of
this. You may feel a persistent instability
in your stomach, or your diaphragm labours,
or you are constricted in your chest or
neck, etc. Of course, seek medical advice

accordingly. But also, be aware that Self
may be 'presenting' in your physicality to
substantiate its position. It is, therefore,
important that Self's role be acknowledged
and that *everything* it promotes in attention
is perceived as an act of protection.
Subsequently meditation becomes
instrumental. Bring the dis-*ease* in your
body into attention and thank Self for its
efforts.

Aoife: How are objects 'dissolved' again?

Dad: Everything comes from consciousness. In
this way there is only consciousness.
Consciousness must be revealed. It is not
achieved or manifested; it is *realised* as
having always been. Meditation can give you
glimpses of consciousness, in which
everything dissolves; the more time spent in
this aware state the more you sense its
pervasiveness. Remember, you cannot be *made*
one-with-everything because everything *is*
one. With meditation you can sense the
oneness, it is then impossible to 'remove'
any item, etc. It is impossible because
there are no individual items; the
realisation of this is the 'dissolving'.

Aoife: So, *oneness* is the key to awakening.

Dad: A 'key' is an *item*. Any objectification
is an act of Self and obscures awareness.
The pursuit of awakening is a contradiction:
you do not drink algebra. Self is a powerful
objectify-er. This approach allows you to
define Self so it can be demoted.

Aoife: So, I must be in the pursuit of
nothing?

Dad: No-*thing* is the default. Some-*thing* is Self, to be used when required. Unfortunately, most people feel Self is their default state. To target *nothing* is to objectify it. There is no-thing to pursue.

Aoife: Why is my awakening not sustainable?

Dad: Self will promote anything rendered by the imagination consistent with its needs. In other words, Self will find a way to objectify your *awakening*. First, do not despise Self for doing this. Second, understand the implication for the story the mind tells itself.

Aoife: Which is?

Dad: It is because of an interruption to the story the mind is telling that you had an awakening experience. Self is a protection tool. It identifies the maintenance of your social viability as the best means for *protecting* the 'being' you are. In this way, it makes the world appear substantive. In doing so, it relies on the imagination's ability to render *everything.* Essentially, Self has at its disposal a never-ending supply of promotable items.

Aoife: So, it is always promoting something?

Dad: Yes. It determines what to promote as the story the mind tells itself changes. In other words, Self *expects* the mind to keep the narrative flowing. Protecting the 'being' is of paramount importance, therefore, Self *must* perceive the narrative. When there is an interruption to the story

Self dissolves; and literally, the essential you is *revealed*.

Aoife: However?

Dad: Indeed. The subsequent *awakening* is temporary and will last for as long as it takes for the mind to reboot. In this way, Self is seeking to provide the mind with an item. Self is vigilant. Therefore, it will attempt to itemise something associated with the awakening.

Aoife: Why?

Dad: Given its protective responsibilities, Self is determined to control any *thing* that effects the telling of the story the mind creates. The beauty of a flower may have impressed you to the extent that it interrupted the story the mind is telling. You experience a micro-awakening; they are frequent but not understood by most people. Self will then itemise the flower; its *impact* dimension will then 'belong' to Self.

Aoife: But Self promoted the flower initially?

Dad: It was promoted because it was immersive. The imagination-rendering-Self-promoting process can be short-circuited when the stimulus is immersive. In other words, rendering and promotion become one act, or autonomic. Our sensors will trigger this overriding effect. In other words, forceful stimuli will be instantly promoted. This is why traumatic events can sometimes trigger a momentary feeling of absence or deep calm.

Aoife: How does the mind know to change the story it tells?

Dad: Because of the data promoted by Self.

Aoife: But Self relies on the story?

Dad: Yes. It is a reciprocating loop. The feedback oscillates between the mind and Self. Not unlike the imagination echo-*rendering* external and internal data. In other words, it is a cycle-informing-cycle that is imperfectly closed.

Aoife: So, permanently interrupting the story is awakening?

Dad: No. You cannot permanently interrupt anything. What you are seeking is revealed. It is there where mind is not.

Aoife: Mind-blind?

Dad: Yes. Awareness is sustained directly. Go in the *direction* of where you are; it is revealed.

Aoife: Consciousness?

Dad: Yes. Everything has its source. What you are seeking *is* the source; it is the only constant.

Aoife: So, I should Be aware of Self being *over* vigilant?

Dad: Hypervigilance is a characteristic of a domineering Self. Hypervigilant people are suffering and latently long for relief. They

have a sophisticated understanding of ego,
but a perception of Self with a blind-spot.
Self is powerfully protective. It learns
survival by gazing into the mirror that is
the mind. The mind fulfils the needs of Self
by showing to it that which it is unable to
momentarily discern. The mind, however, has
no means for distinguishing the difference
between real and imagined threats; the
imagination substantiates *all* data the mind
receives. Therefore, as the mind reflects
Self, Self must also inform the story the
mind tells with greater sensitivity. Self
can do this by allowing the 'observer' to
define the *true* nature of a perceived
threat.

Aoife: What is the blind-spot?

Dad: The recession of awareness relative to
levels of stress. It is the momentary
blindness to *presence*. It is as if the third
umpire 'observer' is being ignored.
Hypervigilance is important when the
Sabretooth Tiger is stalking your tribe.
Hypervigilance is, therefore, a response to
immersive data.

Aoife: How do I relieve hypervigilance?

Dad: Do not devalue presence. Presence *is*
awareness and we know it as the 'observer'.
Remind Self that it is *known*, thank it for
its vigilance and step *out* of the moment and
ask essential questions.

Aoife: Such as - what is the threat to life?

Dad: Yes.

Aoife: What is suffering?

Dad: It is a response to injustice. You suffer when you ask 'why me?' And when you perceive the unanswerable nature of that question to be unfair.

Aoife: Is it unfair?

Dad: All suffering is made of two parts 1. asking 'why me' and 2. expecting an answer. There is no answer for the 'why me' question; it is perplexing, not unjust. The Subsequent astonishment resides within the domain of Self to resolve.

Aoife: Why?

Dad: Astonishment describes an *authentic priming to learn* because it is enabled by the observer point of view. It is awareness engaging in the lesson taught by *now*. However, astonishment informed by injustice is social viability compromising; Self will then seek to objectify.

Aoife: Objectify what?

Dad: The source of the injustice. Self will be unable to promote anything in attention; suffering manifests when there is no clear blame *target*. 'Why me?' will then be promoted by Self.

Aoife: How?

Dad: Remember, *everything* is rendered by the imagination. The thought 'why me?' will be itemised. It may appear in your mind's eye as a cacophony of images, etc. The data will be unstable as Self seeks to attach it to a cause, or in other words, seeks to allocate blame.

Aoife: What then?

Dad: Self promotes this 'unstable' data, it will inform the story the mind tells itself and Self will begin to disconnect from reality. It will be as if the question 'why me?' festers in attention and appear to be indissoluble. It is painful and encourages the mind to tell a story that encourages Self to allocate blame.

Aoife: How do I dissolve the 'why me?' blockage?

Dad: Separate the parts of suffering. 'Why me?' is an item focused question, change it to 'why?'. *Why* is the beginning of the Self inquiry journey; ask *why* with an authentic sense of inquiry and bravery.

Aoife: And the second part?

Dad: Expecting and not receiving an answer to the 'why me?' question appears perplexing; let it become astonishment. Once you have removed the *me* from the 'why me?' question then astonishment is no longer tethered to the desire to allocate blame. Astonishment is then free to manifest as an indicator of authentic inquiry; because of the Self inquiry, you will be amazed at the pervasive nature of Self. Amazement acknowledged from the *observer* position is astonishment. In this way, amazement is befuddling, and astonishment is the recognition of wonder as a means for further inquiry.

Aoife: What are control freaks?

Dad: They are *controlled*. Some people actively promote in their attention the idea that their controlling nature is a stable, innate, integral personality trait. Essentially, they are refusing to use their *own* tools to manage an unpredictable world, instead they force others to use their tools to make the world *appear* more predictable. It is difficult for a controlling personality to *step-back* from this dependency on others. It means Self would have to promote *thought*-items such as - why can't I manage instability? The tendency to be 'controlling' is not innate, it is learnt: *No trait is entirely innate*. The desire to dominate is promoted by Self for a reason. If the source of it is not determined the Self informed by the need to control will experience the failure of its duty.

Aoife: How is the source of it determined?

Dad: The *desire-to-control*, like anything promoted by Self, is a rendered item. It must be allowed to 'sit' in attention prior to its promotion. The 'observer' we *essentially* are, is then able to *acknowledge* it. In other words, the 'observer' makes the rendering available to the imagination 'again'. In this way the 'observer' perspective can be understood as a *sixth* sense. Most people *move* unwittingly, between a state of being *driven* by Self and the 'observer' state. Remember: *My approach does not inhibit this movement; it helps you understand when and how it happens.* The 'observer' is not informed by the story the mind tells. It therefore can only *see* items for what they are. In this instance the *perspective* viewpoint provided by the 'observer' *repackages* the 'control' trait into something more isolated. This principle is known as 'getting perspective' on something. The controlling personality very rarely moves into the 'observer' state. They are unable to experience the joyous nature of its stability; instead, they are *controlled* by Self. Consider: *We all have the desire to control some part of our lives.* In meditation we can *audit* our resistance to change; we can determine to what extent we rely on or manipulate others to maintain that resistance.

Aoife: So, do not force Self to *not* change.

Dad: Yes, Self must adapt or *vary*, that is its purpose. The 'observer', however, is not changeable; it is a third umpire.

Aoife: And we must 'build'?

Dad: Yes. Do not focus on destroying the parts of reality you cannot manipulate and then force others to maintain the vacuum it creates; it is impossible. Maintain a sense of community; an unfulfilled ego self-destructs, it is logical. 'Control' the construction of community, not the constriction of it.

Aoife: How do psychopaths *use* personality?

Dad: They see it as something they must and can 'design'. They are *observers* of Self and this gives them the ability to shape it. But they are powering Self with an unsophisticated appreciation of ego. They develop Self later in life, past a point where Self can acquire a full complement of tools. Their Self-development was delayed due to attachment issues; there was no genuine connection made with a mentor. So, the number of tools available is limited and they will pick and choose them based on reward. Therefore, they will only master tools for which there is the greatest social benefit; they may appear charming and affable. However, because no proper attachment was formed, this 'likeable' *display* works like a disguise to hide the truth: *They are ashamed of their inadequately formed Self even though they cannot perceive the nature of the inadequacy entirely.* This 'likeability' is also designed to manipulate others towards filling the attachment need; they become controlling. Or they want to literally 'possess' others. Their ego is never able to acquire a 'build' dimension because their collection of tools was developed at a stage when dependency need was unfulfilled. Children are dependant and their ego works to energise a trial-and-error approach to Self-development; their *errors* allow their guardians to provide social guidance. Ultimately a healthy ego will learn to 'build' internal *and* external structures as modelled by its guardians. If, however, a dependency need is never fulfilled and attachment is not formed, an ego may never develop external awareness: *The ego will be 'trapped' in protection mode and will only*

know how to 'build' internal structures.
Because of an intense, but not fully
understood, attachment need these
'structures' can appear to work very well
socially. But once dependency begins to form
problems arise. Obsession behaviours emerge
as management strategies as the ego attempts
to fill the attachment void.

Aoife: Is attachment essential?

Dad: Attachment is essential to the
development needs of a child, so much so,
that any distraction that removes attention
from the child during the acquisition phase
will cause the child distress. The child may
then develop an attachment deficiency
informed by attention-seeking.

Aoife: I sometimes feel like my attention
'light' flickers; it cannot *focus.*

Dad: Remember: *The true nature of attention
never changes; it is a streetlight that
'receives' items into it.* Attention
defocusing is best described as Self
zealously over-promoting.

Aoife: What happens then?

Dad: If Self promotes *everything* in
attention the mind is unable to tell a
cohesive story. Consider: *Stressful or
traumatic evets are automatically promoted
by Self. The nature of the event may
prohibit the looping of that data into the
story the mind is telling. Self relies on
the story the mind is telling to determine
what it promotes. Therefore, Self my over-*

*promote and make everything that comes into
attention vivid.*

Aoife: The mind is overwhelmed?

Dad: Yes. Therefore, it is important to
develop a sense of the 'observer',
meditation helps.

Aoife: I do not remember developing
attachment?

Dad: This is the advantage psychopaths have.
They are more directly able to manipulate
their Self to adapt to the needs of others;
they acquired their tools later in life.
You, however, acquired Self in infancy; you
were less cognisant. It means you risk
losing perspective on Self as you mature;
that is why I am having this 'talk' with
you. Ok, so you do not remember acquiring
your Self-tools which means you are not a
psychopath. Psychopaths use Self with more
control, but they have significantly less
tools available.

Aoife: What should I be wary of?

Dad: Someone who 'defends' their position by
making you an integral part of *their* story.

Aoife: Some people are very defensive?

Dad: It is difficult to talk to the
'defender'. *Defender* is the name given to a
person who is forcing Self to highlight in
attention information needed to defend its
position.

Aoife: What position?

Dad: Its social viability.

Aoife: But?

Dad: Yes. Some people are so defensive it compromises their social viability; or so it appears: *A highly defensive person is presenting a 'rationed' set of personality traits (self-tools).*

Aoife: Rationed?

Dad: Yes, they are presenting a personality that consists of only those characteristics necessary to maintain the *status* of Self. They do this because ego is putting aside, any sense of community. That is why it is impossible to rationalise with a defender; balanced perspectives require an expansive sense of ego. People with strident political views often become defenders; they will not hear an opposing point of view. It does not mean however, that your point-of-view is unable to be heard.

Aoife: What do you mean?

Dad: When you are speaking to a *defender* you are being heard by more than the defender they *are*. Imagine, if you will, that you are speaking to a 'defender' but you are also being heard by the 'survivor' aspect of their Self simultaneously. In other words, Self cannot promote a defensive personality and ignore data instrumental to its survival.

Aoife: How is that achieved?

Dad: You say certain things to the survivor
they essentially are and ignore the defender
they are temporarily displaying.

Aoife: What 'certain thing' will I say?

Dad: Everyone desires to receive information
essential to the survival of their Self.
What might that information be?

Aoife: Anything relating to social
viability?

Dad: Yes, but from a *healthy* understanding
of social viability perspective. *"Your role
in this
community/process/exploration/venture/etc is
important and I need your help."* Take a
moment to reflect upon this scripting.
Regardless of its immediate effectiveness,
the part of it that cannot be *unheard* by
Self is the dependence dimension.
Essentially, I am asking you to imagine that
an aspect of Self is always 'listening' from
behind the scenes; it is facilitated by the
imagination.

Aoife: what do you mean by 'dependence
dimension'?

Dad: In any social setting Self cannot
ignore an opportunity to be validated. The
less energy it appears to cost the mind and
body the more likely it is that Self will
accept some dependency. In other words, ego
wants to be relied upon to power Self
towards a diverse appreciation of its
objective.

Aoife: What other scripting can I use?

Dad: Accept the principle and determine your own approach; be genuine.

Aoife: Can you clarify, what is a direct approach to Self-mastery?

Dad: Accept that love and hate, anger, and forgiveness, etc exist at the same time. It may appear as if feelings have timelines; one must end before another can manifest - not true. Remember: *The rainbow is made up of all colours; they are 'available' on the spectrum in equal measure.*

Aoife: So, I can 'directly' replace one feeling with another?

Dad: No. Understanding that Self promotes items in attention means you can 'directly' inform what is promoted. Or in other words, Self can *relearn* what to promote. This relearning can be instantaneous; any promotion can be reassessed in terms of social viability at any time.

Aoife: How?

Dad: Be the 'observer'. Practice *revealing* the 'observer' perspective through meditation and by asking the question — what is the 'thoughtless' me.

Aoife: Thoughtless?

Dad: The sense of your 'being' you experience in the space between your thoughts is constant. Develop your sense of it, it is the gateway to the 'observer' perspective.

Aoife: The 'observer' perspective is the getting-of-perspective?

Dad: Yes.

Aoife: So, I cannot shortcut processing emotions?

Dad: No, they must be 'looked' at. The imagination will place items into attention and Self must 'promote' items that attract processing potential. Remember: *Self is seeking social validation, which is best achieved by displaying to others its ability to process data towards the construction of community.* If you try *not* to process, in effect, you are trying to reduce entropy; it is impossible. The imagination makes *everything* available in attention. Do not change what gets promoted, change *why*.

Aoife: So, feelings are processors?

Dad: Once they are made part of the story. Feelings are used by Self to inform the story the mind is telling; Self provides the parts for the *processor* and the mind assembles it.

Aoife: How do I organise the objects of my attention?

Dad: Good question. Appreciate this 'talk' and understand the purpose of Self, the ego, attention, and consciousness. Define your Self tools, audit their purposefulness and master them. Understand that the imagination renders everything before it appears in attention. Accept that the *rendering* is

making an illusionary world appear
'substantive'. Accept that emotions are like
the colours of the rainbow one bleeds into
the other; in infinite parallel.

Aoife: Are we alone in the universe?

Dad: All 'life' in the universe is a
dumpster fire, burning the waste of the
cosmos. I imagine any agent of entropic
processing corelating on another planet
would not be a fan of reality TV.

Aoife: Does God exist?

Dad: Love exists and is a way of describing
the unity that is consciousness. God can be
understood as the imagination working to
make everything in the 'now' substantive. In
other words, God is the *now*.

Aoife: Should I fear death?

Dad: Does water fear evaporation?

Aoife: I suspect not?

Dad: Then do not fear. Fear *is* death.

Aoife: What do I do now?

Dad: Reflect: *Like the 'wedge' app on your
phone, appreciate it for its silliness. But
if you literally put your phone under the
wobbly leg of the café table the screen will
crack.*

Aoife: Anything else?

Dad: The universe is music. Consciousness
fundamental to the universe is an eternal
hum from a bass amp. The crackles and pops
are universes bursting into life and
decaying. And laughter is the national
anthem of the united-state-of-presence;
laughter is consciousness bubbling to the
surface to share a piece of infinity.

www.ingramcontent.com/pod-product-compliance
Lightning Source LLC
Chambersburg PA
CBHW032114280326
41933CB00009B/830